DISCOVER HOW TO MAINTAIN YOUR BRAIN PLASTICITY FOR LIFE.

THE NEW AMAZING FRONTIER OF **HOPE**.

# BRAIN
# WELLNESS

## THE SECRETS FOR LONGEVITY

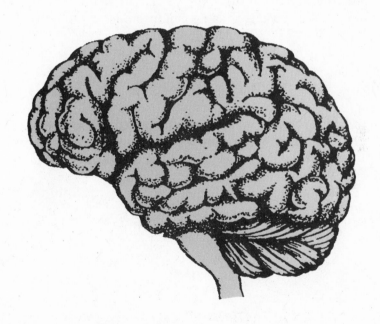

# Gary Anaka
## Brain Coach

Published in Canada in 2009 by
Portal Press
105-1470 Pennyfarthing Dr.
Vancouver BC  V6J 4Y2
hgreavesster@gmail.com

Anaka, Gary 1948
Brain Wellness The Secrets For Longevity

Every effort has been made to trace the critical source of text
and other material. Where the attempt has been unsuccessful,
the publisher would be pleased to hear from copyright holders
to rectify any errors or omissions.

ISBN  978-0-921138-02-0




Editorial Coordination: Howard Greaves
Page Layout: Alison Cole, Intelliga Productions
Artist: Danielle Gauthier
Printed in Canada

# CONTENTS

## Chapter 8  Brain Compatible Lifestyles..........................137

# DISCLAIMER

This book contains the ideas, thoughts and opinions of the author. It is based upon many years of ongoing training, study and teaching in the new exciting field of Applied Educational Neuroscience. It is intended for educational purposes only. This book is not a substitute for the medical recommendations of professional health-care providers. There are no prescriptions for medical treatment of any kind. The reader is solely responsible if he or she chooses to do anything based on what is written in this book. This book is meant to be a catalyst to help you educate yourself about how to live in a more healthy, brain compatible way.

# ACKNOWLEDGEMENTS

I started working in the field of Applied Educational Neuroscience in 1997. I wish to thank all the endless numbers of people of all ages, all walks of life and all professions who have consistently given positive feedback to my presentations about brain health and wellness and how the brain learns. Thank you to Howard Greaves for his great support and enthusiasm for a future healthy, intelligent society. Thank you to Danielle Gauthier for the artwork. And a special, heartfelt thanks to Maureen, my wife, for her endless invaluable support in producing this book.

THIS HUMBLE BOOK IS

DEDICATED TO

REKINDLING THE

HUMAN SPIRIT

THROUGH

BRAIN WELLNESS

# *BRAIN WELLNESS*

## IS A BOOK FOR YOU IF...

You are worried about:
- always being mentally exhausted or have low energy
- losing or misplacing things
- dozing off in meetings or in the afternoon
- not being as sharp as you used to be
- getting old before your time

You would like to get better at:
- remembering things, places, events, and names
- being more productive, creative, and useful
- having full brain power all day long
- keeping your perfectly fine brain working

You want to:
- support and learn more about yourself
- avoid the perils of multitasking
- avoid cognitive decline
- eliminate the hazards of potential brain burn out
- live with successful cognitive aging

**YOUR BRAIN HAS UNLIMITED POTENTIAL**

**FIND OUT HOW TO UNLEASH IT**

# INTRODUCTION

Your health is the most treasured possession you have. At the center of that reality is your body's single most crucial organ – your **brain**. Your brain is your true center of your sense of self. Your brain sustains your quality of life. It is the organ of learning, working and relating to everything and everyone in your life. If you are not well, your brain is not well. Who wouldn't want insights on brain wellness?

I am a teacher. I have worked as a Learning Assistance Specialist in High School for over 30 years. My particular area of expertise is how the brain learns. Not so much from the technical, scientific point of view, but rather from a totally practical "how can I help you to learn this" perspective. I have come to see through the years, that children and adults are now having more difficulty learning, focusing, paying attention, solving problems and remembering things. There are many, many reasons for this but the bottom line is that more and more people are experiencing brain problems. I am not a neuroscientist, nor a medical doctor, nor do I have a PhD: I am a very concerned public educator and I want to educate you. Without knowledge we can't progress intelligently in our lives. Knowledge is needed or we remain ignorant about why our lives aren't working so well.

I am presently a middle-aged baby boomer. I experienced a very unhealthy childhood. As a result, my personal health has always been a top priority for me. Today it is even more so, especially my brain health. Society in general seems to conclude that once you pass youth and early adulthood, your brain experiences an inevitable decline. Everyone loses brainpower. That's the way it is. That dynamic, zestful brain power of youth is gone forever. Life becomes progressively duller. Generally, it is conceded, that brain degeneration is our fate.

For some, that most scary and dark condition of **senility** looms ahead. The fear is that the longer you live, the greater the likelihood is of getting a disease like Alzheimer's or Parkinson's. I am happy to share with you a more optimistic and hopeful reality: **IT DOESN'T HAVE TO HAPPEN!** I personally have no interest in brain degeneration now or in the future. I hope you don't either. These negative realities can be avoided. A rebirth in brainpower is possible!

## NEUROSCIENCE HAS ANSWERS

In 1950, there were only a few hundred neuroscientists in the entire world. Today there are over 32,000. Neuroscience is the hottest science on earth. Imagine the fame and fortune for the scientist who invents a remedy to help you recover your memory. If a scientist could find a cure for Alzheimer's disease, what a great contribution to humanity that would be. Imagine the interest and hope from all of humanity for knowledge and understanding about how to live with a perfectly healthy brain throughout your entire lifetime. We are living in an exciting era in history when these things are no longer considered impossible or even bizarre.

Neuroscience is really in the Stone Age. Virtually everything we know about the human brain has come to us in the last 20 years. The 1990's was the decade of the brain that opened up many new frontiers and great discoveries with promises of more to come.

I am presenting a simple overview of the most significant brain research. It's not possible to talk about every aspect of brain research and, of course, there are exceptions for everything. The information presented to you in this book is now common knowledge. The hope is that you will share with your family and friends. Everyone will benefit.

I am a brain coach and my message is simple. I wrote this book in plain language with a common sense approach. It's a non-academic and non-technical self-help book. I feel that there is a huge need to educate all members of society.

Hopeful, optimistic news is reaching us that you should be aware of. There are lots of ways to make your brain better. By your own efforts you can improve your brain's performance. Cognitive decline does not have to be your future. Through knowledge and understanding, you can tune up your brain, grow your brain, avoid brain dysfunction, and slow down your brain from aging. If you have a good brain right now, keep it that way. The future health and longevity of your brain is in your hands. As you age wouldn't you want to be more than just alive and getting by? Why not live well into old age and **NOT REGRET IT**.

Reading and applying *BRAIN WELLNESS THE SECRETS FOR LONGEVITY* will get you started on that path. Enjoy your journey!

# BRAIN

# DEGENERATION IS

# EASIER

# TO PREVENT THAN

# REPAIR

# CHAPTER 1

# Is Your Brain Aging Too Quickly?

In the past, brain scientists were rather pessimistic about preventing brain aging. With great advances in biological research and computer technology today, there is greater hope to avoid mental decline in old age. But, first it's important to ask yourself the question "Will my brain go the distance?"

# 1.1  THE SIGNS

Do you ever experience this?

You are walking down the street in your hometown. A person approaches who is quite familiar to you. In fact, you have known this person for years but just cannot remember his name. Or, when introduced to a stranger, you shake their hand and immediately forget their name. The important factor is how often these lapses occur: once in a while or everyday? How about forgetting appointments, misplacing your keys, not remembering all the things you went to the store to buy, or having trouble recalling an everyday object. Are you a person who needs five or six pairs of reading glasses because you misplace them all the time? Have you ever bought a coffee, placed it on the roof of your car and driven off leaving it up there? On occasion this happens to all of us. You need to honestly ask yourself, is my memory gradually getting worse as I get older? **Memory loss is one of the first signs of brain aging**.

Do you get tired more easily at work or at home? Sometimes you might nod off in the late afternoon or even have trouble staying awake. Your mental stamina is not what it used to be. Years ago, it was easy for you to concentrate for hours on end. Now, it is more of a challenge. Mental exhaustion just seems to be a way of life. Simple math calculations in your head are more difficult to do. Perhaps you rely more on a calculator. Often times you may find yourself just staring blankly at the computer for 5 to 10 minutes. Learning something new or taking on a new project is difficult because you are just too tired. Your thinking may be slowing down. It is more than likely that your brain can no longer process information as fast as it used to. Unfortunately, even though your brain knows the answer, you can't get the information out as quickly as you used to. **A tired brain is the second indicator of an aging brain.**

I often experienced this situation at work in my classroom during my last years of teaching. My classroom usually held students in it who were in grades 8, 9, 10, 11, and 12. Thus, I was hopping from student to student, subject to subject, grade level to grade level continually, day in and day out for years. Typically, after helping a student, I would get up and walk across the room, stop dead in my tracks and not have a clue as to why I went to the other side. In just a few seconds I had gotten totally off task. Lost it! Complicating this frustrating occurrence, my concentration and mental performance were compromised. It became harder and harder to do many things at once and my job became more stressful as time went by.

On the other hand, the students I was teaching could listen to music, talk to each other, and do their assignments all at the same time with no problem. The students had a young brain and could easily multitask. Older brains have trouble absorbing tons of information quickly. An older brain can't handle information overload as well as a younger brain can. **Older brains experience this commonplace failure in multitasking. This is often another sign of brain aging.**

I hear lots of jokes about failing memories and 'senior moments' especially from middle aged and older people. People often laugh at these memory lapses. The reality is that we treat these experiences lightly because we are really nervous and fearful deep down inside. It's not funny if it is happening to you, or your partner, or a friend all the time. The signs described above: brain overload, a tired brain, memory loss or troubles multitasking are usually normal signs of aging. People naturally get mentally slower over the years. A midlife slow down is to be expected. That is the reality for most of us.

However, not too many of us are conscious of the aging process of our body, let alone the aging of our brain. Continuous memory loss, brain fatigue, mental exhaustion and a quickening loss of cognitive faculties are NOT normal. These are warning signs. Something is not right.

If you feel that you are 'losing it' then that's exactly what may be happening. You may be wearing out your brain parts at an accelerated pace. Your brain is flesh and blood. It won't last forever. It must be clearly understood, that wearing your brain out is a real possibility.

A prematurely deteriorating brain is a tragedy. If these experiences are continually part of your life, then WAKE UP! PAY ATTENTION! There are no magic pills to get your memory back. There are no magic pills to restore an exhausted worn out brain. You cannot buy a new brain. Your lifestyle may be promoting and fast forwarding the downfall of your own brain.

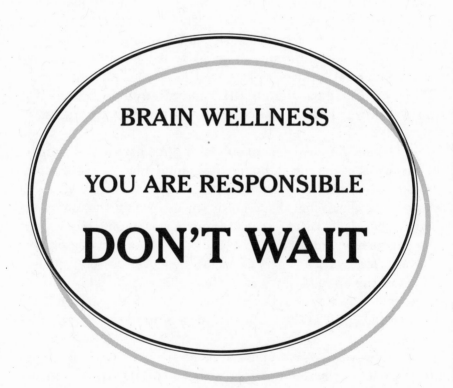

**BRAIN WELLNESS**

**YOU ARE RESPONSIBLE**

# DON'T WAIT

# 1.2 WHY YOUR BRAIN IS AGING

Why is your brain aging? The answer is not because of a single phenomenon or a single process. There are many theories about brain aging. However, here is a simplified overview of the main dilemma.

**After age 30, the brain begins to shrink**. The total volume of brain tissue slowly decreases with daily wear and tear. There is a reduction in the number of brain cells called neurons. You literally have billions of neurons in your brain. There is enough to last your whole lifetime. But, the problem is how they change over time. Connections between them are very important to maintain. Losing the connectors between these cells is the real problem. As well, the covering around the neurons can deteriorate. These are the reasons for the decrease in brain volume, which occurs with normal aging.

When this deterioration occurs, **the electrical activity of the brain slows down**. The signals between neurons get slower and slower. One very noticeable result is that, with advancing age, paying attention becomes harder. The filters that block out sensory noise and constant stimulation begin to falter. The brain has to deal with more distractions and registers more confusion, thus making it harder to stay on task.

**The brain produces less neurotransmitters (chemicals) as we age**. This sometimes accounts for why people get more irritable and grumpy with age. As well, genetics play a significant role for some people. How well you age depends on your genes. Finally, if your body is healthy, your brain is healthy. If your body is sick, then your brain is likely to be sick too. The brain is not isolated from the body. A deterioration in bodily health means deterioration in brainpower too.

As you age, it is obvious that **the brain has fewer resources**. Perhaps the major player in brain aging is a lack of blood flow to the brain. Less oxygen is getting to the neurons. This also means that the waste products can't be carried away. Without a constant supply of oxygen, brain aging and disease are sure to come.

**The older you are the more vulnerable your brain is.** If some of the aging signs are part of your life, realize that they can lead to more serious problems. Accelerated brain aging leaves your brain vulnerable to more serious neurological diseases.

It is true that the aging brain does slow down naturally. But, neuroscientists are now saying that you can control your own destiny more than you think. The brain's neurons have to be supported by an intelligent life style. They need to be cared for if you expect them to work well for you. They need to be protected and nurtured if you want to maintain a high quality of life as you age. Your brain does not have to succumb to the ravages of time. Your brainpower does not have to decrease as the years go by. You can stay mentally sharp as you age.

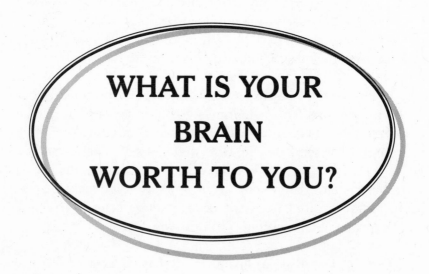

# WHAT IS YOUR BRAIN WORTH TO YOU?

# CHAPTER 2

# Brain Coaching

All sorts of activities and games get support from coaches. The most wonderful game of all, the game of life, needs a coach too. However, society in general is not prepared to handle the newest version of this game – longevity. The health of the body has been prolonged but what about the health of the mind? Living to a very old age is a real possibility for many people but you have to have a healthy brain to enjoy it with. To play the Brain Wellness game and win, you need a brain coach.

# 2.1 GET A COACH

Many of us have had a coach at one time or another in our lives. Coaches offer services needed to gain new skills. They expand our awareness, provide leadership and expertise. So where in the world can you find a brain coach? That's easy! **YOU!**

Yes, be your own brain coach. Don't rely on anyone else to figure your brain out for you. Become your own expert. Maybe you and I will never completely understand what goes on in there. But, that is a good reminder that we don't know much about ourselves. The motto from the ancient Greek Civilization is still relevant today – **"Man, know thyself"**.

This is a very radical approach indeed. Our society is programmed for something or someone to bail us out all the time. If something is wrong, we automatically look for outside help or a pill for our problems. Well, don't wait passively as the years pass and your lights get dimmer. Don't expect your Doctor or a prescription to save you when you finally realize you have a problem. You have to **act now**, especially if you are over the age of 30. This is a huge dilemma and you don't have many options. Every one of us is at risk from cognitive decline, no exceptions.

Time to start some brain training. What could be more vital to your life, your relationships, your children, and your community? Take confidence in what the thousands of scientific articles and research findings are saying about the many ways there are to build or maintain your brain. Of course, there is no one single path to follow. We are all unique and diverse in our own ways. So, the need is to find your own remedies. Make **personal choices** to suit your needs and lifestyle. Individualize your efforts to obtain the best results for you based on what is currently known about the brain.

Let's start. Your basic equipment is your brain. Be grateful you have a brain. Believe in your brain. Believe in yourself too. That fantastic brain of yours is always changing and growing. Both of these realities are built in features that are designed to support you for the long haul. If your brain can direct its own future, then why can't you?

Preventing dementia is like a numbers game: you have to play all the variables to win. You will live many more years, so plan ahead. Set some goals. Work out a game plan. Create new paradigms for each future stage of your life. Your life is in control when you control your life.

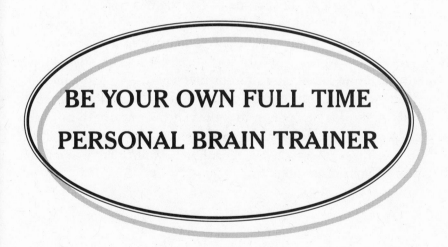

**BE YOUR OWN FULL TIME PERSONAL BRAIN TRAINER**

## 2.2 SELF-ASSESSMENT

Think back. Do you have the same brainpower that you had 5 or 10 years ago? Are the abilities that you have always taken for granted slipping away? If you can honestly say that you are not as sharp as you used to be, then you could be **right**. The best assessment is a self-assessment.

It makes sense to recognize problems early. Lapses in memory are normal and of course get more frequent as we age unless they become **increasingly** more frequent. This may not be normal. It may be time to get some help. Other signals to be aware of are mood swings, changes in sleeping patterns, difficulties with balance or just getting around. Be proactive and read the warning signs.

This book is not just about getting new information. It's about motivating you to **take action**. It's presenting you with a new awareness. If you are already a motivated person, you are well on your way. If you are not sure, get lots of advice from many different people in different fields because no one individual has all the solutions for you. Team up with your partner, family members or friends to help you become the best coach that you can be. Make some good choices and come up with a brain wellness plan today. After all, you want to have a passing grade on your assessment.

## 2.3 WHAT'S AHEAD

The overall directions we are taking are optimistic indeed. The future holds much promise and hope. Based on today's needs, therapies will be fantastic. Imagine treatments to actually prevent or stop brain deterioration, overcome alcoholism or drug addiction. Imagine better healing techniques for depression or mental illness. Doctors may have the potential of restoring health anywhere in the body with stem cells. Perhaps the brain could be stimulated to replace its own cells.

But, please do not wait for medical miracles. There will be no miracle tonics for the brain for a long time to come. The field of neuroscience is young. There is every reason to believe these remedies will happen, but don't hold your breath waiting for them.

In the immediate future, I see clearly that the brain wellness movement will start to snowball. Brain Health could easily become a trillion dollar industry because our collective brain is going to need a lot of help. Many of the following brain wellness trends will begin to manifest in our society in the very near future. Hyperbaric oxygen tanks will be a common feature in people's homes. Hyperbaric oxygen therapy can boost the level of oxygen in your cells to promote healing. Far infrared saunas will replace conventional saunas and hot tubs. They will become a significant player in personal wellness programs. These saunas provide radiant heat that induces a deep sweat for cleansing and detoxifying the body. More people will be using air filter systems and negative ionizers. In general, people have to be more responsible for their own health and brain wellness.

In addition, Western medicine will have to accept the philosophies and teachings from the East. The fact that the mind can control the body is no longer a mystery. Eastern practices, once considered bizarre, will soon be orthodox.

The Federal and Provincial governments need to consider giving tax breaks to companies and organizations that support the Canadian brain. (No tax on sports equipment, exercise equipment, health foods, health supplements, health books or magazines, for example.)

Finally, a more proactive approach by all levels of government in Canada is needed. Brain problems are real and are increasing dramatically as our population ages. Literally millions are going to be affected. A **'save the Canadian brain'** mass media campaign that pushes Canadians to care for their brains more responsibly can avoid a lot of suffering... and money. The worst fears about pandemics involving mad cow disease, avian flu, West Nile virus, and SARS all combined have killed only a few people in our country. In contrast, the devastating effects of fatal neurological diseases spread like wildfire from coast to coast. There is an incredible growth in the number of people being diagnosed with Alzheimer's or related dementias. Neuroscientists know about it. Public health workers know about it. Sadly, the average man on the street doesn't know or lives his daily life thinking, "It will never happen to me".

What's ahead? Dollars need to be invested in far reaching public education campaigns that eliminate the old myths and make the general public aware of the warning signs. Otherwise sickness, fear, misery and costs are going to skyrocket. Practical ways to save the brain need to be put into action to defend against memory loss, failing minds and the fast approaching wave of brain degeneration.

# 2.4 THE FIGHT OF YOUR LIFE

By nature, the brain's major purpose is to **survive**. Of all the millions of bits of information coming into your brain everyday, anything that affects survival takes priority over everything else. The biggest battle in life then, is to help your brain stay alive and well. By using the scientifically based strategies outlined in this book, you can defend your brain. These options are understandable and reasonable. Put them into action. The brain fitness movement is interesting. Be a part of it. Join up! Fight against memory loss. Fight against brain fog and cognitive decline. They are monsters slowly attacking you. Battle against Alzheimer's disease. The enemies are huge. If you don't pay attention, the very essence of your identity will be stolen from you. Your most valued possession, your optimally functioning brain, could be lost forever. What a catastrophe! What a tragic personal blow not being able to realize your potential as a human being. You can shape your own destiny or destroy your own dignity. **You choose**!

Here is another scourge sweeping our nation from coast to coast: **mediocrity**. Mediocrity sucks! You can argue that some people are born mediocre. I say you can grow out of it! Some people strive to achieve mediocrity. That's an excuse to avoid life. Of course, other people have mediocrity forced upon them. Right. Don't accept that either. Move on. Mediocrity slows and hampers you. Don't be too complacent and let things slide. Why would you let someone else order for you all the time in a restaurant? Why would you let someone else pick your clothes to wear every day? Refusing to make decisions gives away your personal power. Do your own stuff. Mediocrity is a brain losing attitude. Fight it. Avoid stagnation to stay alive.

On another front, you need to fight against gradual brain shrinkage. Every year your brain shrinks a bit. Every year your brain produces fewer neurotransmitters. Every year learning and remembering can become more difficult. Fight against this decline. The average person knows very little about brain wellness. To be honest, just by observing people's behaviour, they are totally unaware of the ordinary things in their lives that take away their brain power, age their brain and leave them defenseless against brain disease.

My greatest recommendation of all is to avoid brain problems before they even start. Why fight if you don't have to? Start by ignoring the aging myths and the decrepit old stereotypes. **Take preventative steps now to avoid future risks.** There won't be any mystical help down the road. You will never regret accepting and integrating some brain smart strategies into your life today. After all, Brain Wellness is a 'do it yourself activity'.

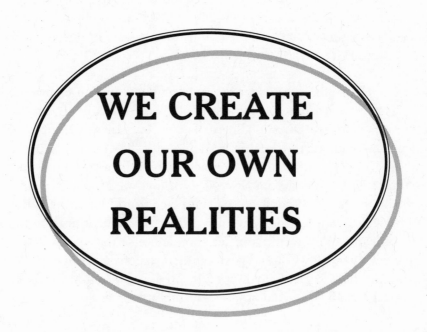

# WE CREATE
# OUR OWN
# REALITIES

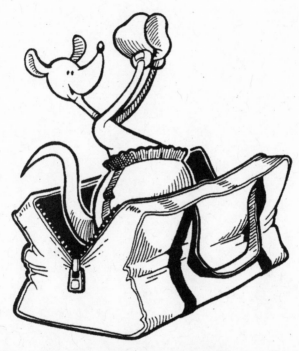

# The Most Important Item In Your Gym Bag Is Your Attitude!

Doug McCallum. Don't Send Your Turkeys to Eagle School, TOOL THYME FOR TRAINERS, 1994.

# Chapter 3

# A Simple Brain Tour

Your brain does a lot of key functions for you. It constantly collects, sorts and circulates information to guide our every action. Knowing how the brain works is critical for your brain wellness program.

Even though I will be outlining parts of the brain separately, they are definitely not separate from each other. Your brain is a complex system. No part of it works in isolation. All the parts work together as a whole unit. Simple tasks like writing with a pen, eating with a fork, solving a puzzle, or talking to a friend require a complex set of interactions between many parts of your brain.

# 3.1  OLD WORN OUT MYTHS

**1.  We are born with a genetically predetermined brain.**
We all have lots of limitations and nothing can be done about it.
The brain is a hardwired black box. You get what you got. This
is simply not true!

**2.  We only use 10% of our brain.** This is also a myth. There
is no scientific data that supports this statement.
Unfortunately, this myth is repeated by the media and society
in general and people believe it. We use all of our brain. That's
why we have one.

**3.  You cannot grow new brain cells.** Brain scientists used
to think that people were born with a fixed number of brain cells
that die out as we got older. It was believed for over 100 years
by neurologists that there was no chance of regeneration. Today
we know that this is simply not true. It is possible to grow new
brain cells well up into old age. That's good news!

**4.  The brain can't change.** For a long time, neuroscientists
believed that once you became an adult, your brain remained
stable for the rest of your life. Then, as the decades passed, the
brain inevitably declined in function and in its structures.
Again, this is no longer thought to be true.

**5.  There is nothing you can do about brain aging.** This out
of date, obsolete assumption should be totally ignored. Brain
integrity can be maintained into old age. There is a lot of
hopeful research and advice being given to us by state of the art
neuroscientists today. Early mental deterioration doesn't have
to be your future. That's today's new reality. Awesome news!

## Neurogenesis: the brain can grow new neurons

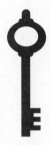 **KEY POINT:** This means that **you** can:

- ☑ grow new brain cells everyday
- ☑ grow new brain cells at any age
- ☑ grow new brain cells until the last day of your life

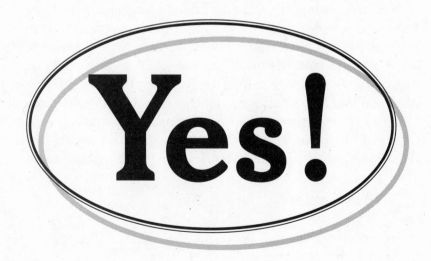

Yes!

## 3.2  BRAIN HEMISPHERES

The brain has two hemispheres: right and left. Raise your arms in front of you and make two fists. Place your fists together. Your two closed fists would be about the same size as your brain. If you open your clenched fists, you would have a right and left hemisphere of equal size!

The CORPUS CALLOSUM (Diagram A) connects the right hemisphere to the left hemisphere. It is a dense band of more than 250 million nerves. Information exchanged between the two hemispheres travels across the corpus callosum.

The function of each hemisphere has literally been debated for centuries. In general, here are the main duties of the left hemisphere: controls the right side of the body, logic, judgments, analysis, literal interpretations, numbers, calculations, and classifies ideas. The main duties of the right hemisphere are: controls the left side of the body, colours, music, visual patterns, images, spatial information, novelty, and intuition. Simply put, the left side is academic and the right side is creative.

These are older theories and are only partially correct. The brain is very complex and complicated. It is true that each hemisphere has specialties, but there is a lot of overlapping. Every thought that the brain has cannot be located in one specific place. Behaviours cannot be located in one specific place either. Music and art, for example, are not just right-brained activities. It is better to take the approach that whatever is happening in the brain is happening throughout the entire brain. The two halves of your brain work in complete partnership.

## Corpus Collosum
**(connects hemispheres)**

**Left Hemisphere**   **Right Hemisphere**

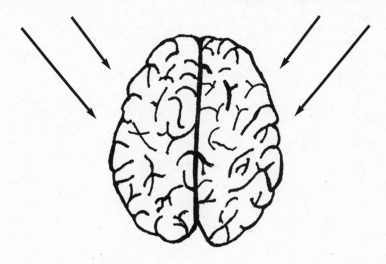

# 3.3 THE CEREBRUM (THE FOUR LOBES)

Most pictures you see of the brain show the folded and grooved CEREBRUM similar to the one on the book cover. It is the largest part of the brain and has been divided into four areas called lobes.

The Frontal Lobe is the area around your forehead. It performs our most complex functions like planning, problem solving, thinking, judgment, creativity and having conversations. It is the most highly developed area of your brain and you will be learning lots about it.

The Parietal Lobe is located on the top, back area of your brain. Its duties consist of sensory and language functions. This part of the brain allows you to focus.

The Temporal Lobes are located around the ears on the right and left side of the brain. Language, speech, hearing, memory and writing occur in this part of the brain.

The Occipital Lobe is in the middle back of the brain. It is responsible for receiving and processing visual information.

- Overlapping does occur between the lobes.

(Diagram B)

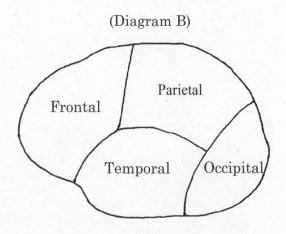

# 3.4 THE MIDDLE BRAIN

This part of the brain (also called the limbic system) is located behind the frontal lobes and in front of the occipital lobe. Here are the key structures that you need to know about.

## Thalamus

This is the brain's relay station and is located at its centre. It acts like a switch. All the information coming into the brain from what we see, hear, feel, touch, taste and smell goes into the Thalamus. Signals are then sent to different parts of the brain for processing.

## Amygdala

The amygdala is an almond-shaped structure located in the middle of the brain. It processes emotions. The amygdala is the fear switch and the key to the fight or flight response.

## Hippocampus

This structure plays a major role in your memory formation. It is critical for learning because it transfers information from short-term memory to long-term memory for storage.

## THE ADULT BRAIN

- weighs approximately 3 pounds or 1.2 kilograms
- is only 2% of your total body weight
- has about 100 billion neurons
- is white, beige and gray in colour
- can easily be cut with a dinner knife

(Diagram C)

# A Medial View Of The Brain

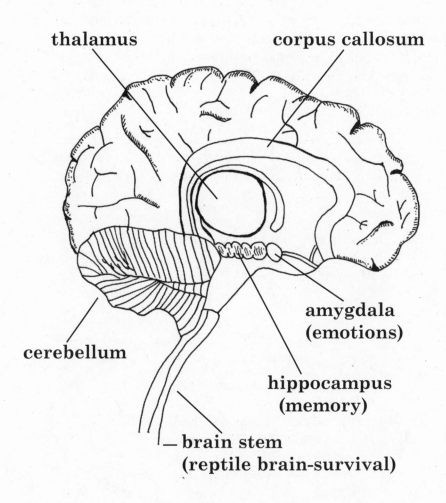

thalamus

corpus callosum

amygdala
(emotions)

cerebellum

hippocampus
(memory)

brain stem
(reptile brain-survival)

# 3.5   THE PREFRONTAL CORTEX
## ('THE CAPTAIN OF THE SHIP')

Place your fingers on your forehead. You have just made contact with 'THE CAPTAIN OF THE SHIP'. The PREFRONTAL CORTEX is the front one-third of your brain, and is the most evolved part. Animals do not have a prefrontal cortex. Therefore, in terms of anatomy, this defines what it means to be a human being.

The prefrontal cortex performs the executive functions of your life. The highest forms of mental activity such as thinking, planning, organizing, judgment, forethought, reasoning, goal setting, concentration, attention span, impulse control, and a whole host of other activities occur here. It allows us to make associations between names and objects. It grants us the ability to express language. Look around you and see all the wonderful things in your life. The 'Captain' supports us to build things, invent things, and create things. It allows us to dream and project into the future. It is what makes us human.

## 3.6  THE CEREBELLUM (THE LITTLE BRAIN)

The CEREBELLUM is located near the brain stem. It is known as the 'little brain'. It is involved in the key activities of body posture, coordination, balance, and muscle function. You couldn't walk across the room without it, nor could you hit a tennis ball or wave to a friend. You can thank your cerebellum for remembering how to ride a bike, drive a car, type on your keyboard or play the piano. The 'little brain' supports you to move and do complex motor activities with little conscious awareness on your part.

There is a HUGE, significant connection between the little brain and the frontal cortex where we do our thinking and learning.

(Diagram D)

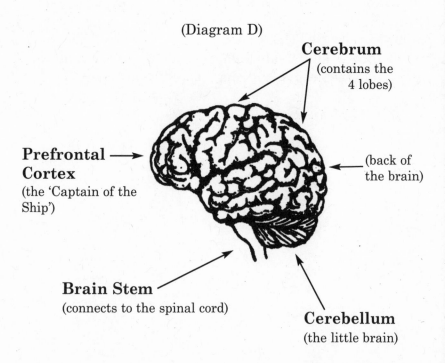

**Cerebrum**
(contains the
4 lobes)

**Prefrontal** ⟶
**Cortex**
(the 'Captain of the
Ship')

(back of
the brain)

**Brain Stem**
(connects to the spinal cord)

**Cerebellum**
(the little brain)

# 3.7 WHAT BRAIN CELLS LOOK LIKE

There are two kinds of brain cells: NEURONS and GLIA. The majority of your brain cells are glia. Glia out number neurons 10 to 1. They are worker cells carrying nutrients, taking away wastes, and helping with the immune system.

NEURONS, on the other hand, give you your brainpower. It is these that you need to know about. Each neuron has its own cell body. Radiating from the cell body are branch-like extensions called DENDRITES. They are like radar antennae constantly picking up signals. From the bottom of the cell body extends one long, thin tail that acts like a telephone line. It is called an AXON. Finally, this axon branches many, many times connecting with other cells through micro gaps called SYNAPSES. Neurons all connect together to form pathways or neural networks.

> **KEY POINT:** Brain aging can be alleviated by knowing how to grow dendrites.

(Diagram E)

## A NEURON

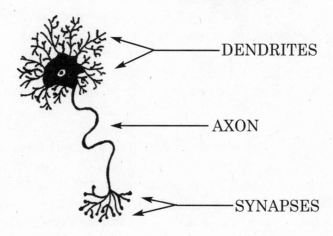

DENDRITES

AXON

SYNAPSES

# 3.8 HOW BRAIN CELLS WORK

You have about 100 billion brain cells. That's good news. These neurons make thousands of connections with other neurons through dendrites. The number of connections neurons can make is unlimited. The more dendrites you have the better it is for you. Neurons continuously fire to generate information. Your neurons are always working, they never sleep.

Absolutely everything you see, do, feel, read, that is literally all human behaviour, can be traced to the communication between neurons. How is this done? Neurons communicate with each other by chemical and electrical signals. The electrical signals travel down the axon to other neurons. Neurons constantly chatter to each other. Your brain is a noisy place.

The axon is insulated by a fatty substance called MYELIN. Myelin helps to speed up electrical transmissions and reduce interference from other reactions. The larger the axon, the more they are myelinated. Lost your keys? Missing something? Myelin has a lot to do with that and your memory. The loss of myelin over time contributes to the loss of memory.

When electrical impulses travel down the axon, they trigger the release of chemicals called NEUROTRANSMITTERS. These neurotransmitters are absorbed by receptor sites in the dendrites of another cell. The release of these chemicals is how the cells talk to each other. Neurotransmitters are the biochemical messengers of the brain. They either stop or start neural activity. These brain chemicals are the highways carrying all your thoughts and feelings.

Once you pass age 30, there are two challenges to be aware of. Firstly, you produce less and less neurotransmitters year after year. Secondly, the number of receptors that take in and release neurochemical messages decreases. Their efficiency also decreases. It is critical to be aware of these realities. There are over 100 neurotransmitters known today. Here are three primary ones.

## Serotonin

Serotonin is the most common and widely studied neurotransmitter. It is your brain's mood regulator. When you are in a good, happy mood your levels of serotonin are up. Ever seen anyone with a glow on his or her face – that's serotonin. It promotes optimism, relaxation, and is required for learning and memory. Low serotonin levels cause us to be anxious, aggressive and depressed. Melatonin is a hormone that is made from serotonin. When melatonin is produced in the brain, it causes us to go to sleep.

## Dopamine

Dopamine is a powerful, common neurotransmitter. It is also involved in producing positive moods or feelings. For example, when your team does well in a game or you win the lottery, you are totally excited. That's dopamine. When you spontaneously do something, that's dopamine. Also, this chemical controls your energy levels: the release of energy, consumption of energy and the production of energy. Finally it plays a role in movement. Parkinson's disease is a severe dopamine deficiency.

## Acetylcholine

Acetylcholine's main function has to do with memory. Your memory circuits won't work without it nor can information be passed through all the brain cells. Aging leads to a decline in acetylcholine. One of the many causes of Alzheimer's disease is a deprivation of this chemical.

One of the major keys to avoiding brain aging is to have knowledge of how to deliberately increase the brain's neurotransmitters. This is not idle speculation. You can influence how well your brain functions through lifestyle changes, food and brain booster supplements.

Here is an example of how neurotransmitters work. You have decided to learn how to juggle. This is a new skill, so when you start to practice your reward system starts to kick in. After the first few practices, the juggling balls actually stay in the air longer and longer. Each success means you feel a little better because you are achieving your goal. Dopamine is released as a reward. When dopamine is released, you feel more self-confident and more self-assured. It is the all time feeling good neurotransmitter. Your feedback system produces the right chemicals when learning a new skill. As well, acetylcholine is released which helps your brain remember how to juggle. More success means more rewards. If you practice with great intensity and really focus you make great changes in the brain. Your brain is switched onto juggling and you feel like a winner!

# Chapter 4

# Brain Basics

On a biological level, it is essential to understand what the brain needs to operate on a moment-to-moment basis. If the essentials aren't supplied, brainpower can't be produced and our potential can't be realized. Today's increasingly complex world forces us to use more and more of our brains. For children, teens, young adults, baby-boomers and seniors these brain basics need to become second nature.

# 4.1 YOUR BRAIN IS AN OXYGEN ADDICT

No oxygen, no brain! Oxygen is the key element needed for your brain to function. Your brain is only 2% of your total body weight but consumes large quantities of oxygen. If it doesn't get a constant supply, it can die within minutes.

Oxygen is a basic element needed to sustain life. It has several main functions including converting carbohydrates, proteins and fats into energy. It cleanses the toxins and cellular waste from the body. It is an energy source for every cell in your body. And most significantly, it is the key element for brain function. Your billions of brain cells produce energy. If the brain cells get an abundance of oxygen they can produce more brainpower for you. Therefore, if the level of oxygenation increases, brain potential and brain function also increase. If you bolster your engine, you can get more horsepower.

Sadly, our modern sedentary lifestyle prevents us from processing enough oxygen. We just take breathing for granted. Thus, our bloodstream can often be oxygen depleted. Oxygen depleted bodies and oxygen depleted brains mean premature aging, less resistance to disease and lowered levels of health and wellbeing. Most people aren't getting enough oxygen.

The answer to this generic problem is obvious. You need to move more. Clean fresh air is essential for the brain's wellbeing. Nature is *the* best place to get it. A regular, systemic and sufficient exercise program is crucial to sustain a healthy brain and to improve neural metabolism. The brain is hungry for oxygen – it is one of the fundamental necessities of the brain. **Lack of oxygen is undoubtedly one of the main reasons for brain deterioration.**

## 4.2 YOUR BRAIN IS MOSTLY WATER

More than any other organ in our bodies, the brain is comprised of mostly water, about 75-80% – the same percentage as our planet. Water is vital to life and vital to your brain. It is the most abundant inorganic substance in the human body.

Water doesn't look like much, but there's no life without it. It won't make you smarter, but it is essential for brain function. Water is essential to life and learning because it is responsible for every biological process, chemical reaction and mechanical action that takes place within our bodies. It is crucial to mental performance.

Every cell in your brain gets oxygen delivered to it by water! The electrical activity across cell membranes cannot occur without water. Water gives us an instant energy boost. Keeping your system hydrated will keep your brain working at optimum efficiency, give you sustained energy and keep you away from stress.

As we age, the total amount of body fluids in us decreases. This means that our circulatory system is very sensitive to changes in water levels. Dehydration becomes easier. Many physicians and scientists are warning that too many of us live in a **partial state of dehydration** or, worse, a **permanent state of dehydration**. This means that the brain is functioning at less than full capacity. Longer times are needed to dispose of wastes. Inadequate levels of water mean electrical problems in the brain. It means more fatigue, apathy, brain fog and a whole host of other undesirable conditions. People of all ages are not drinking enough water in our society today.

**Thirst signals are too late**. Don't wait to get thirsty. You may need water even before you are thirsty. Humans need to drink 1-2 litres a day depending on their weight, their activity and what the weather situation is. That's 8 big glasses.

Sipping water all day long is highly recommended.

So, water is the most sensible drink for you and your brain. Since many people have an unknown dehydration problem, make a new habit. Also, remember that many things people drink are diuretics such as alcohol, coffee, or pop. Diuretics dehydrate your brain. When water levels decrease in the brain, the thirsty signal is sent out. Unfortunately, people continue to drink the same diuretics such as multiple cups of coffee all day long. Drinking water instead, is a much better choice whether you are thirsty or not.

Here are more healthy tips to consider. After drinking a can of beer or a glass of wine, have a glass of water right after. This helps prevent dehydration. You can avoid a big hangover and headache if you drink lots of water after drinking alcohol. This makes good sense. Next, room temperature water is healthier for you than ice water because it does not cool the body's core temperature down. Finally, here's a great tip from Applied Kinesiology. Make a habit of holding water in your mouth for 2 or 3 seconds before swallowing. The water will be kept longer in the intestines and more will be absorbed into the body rather than being passed out of the body.

I no longer drink from my municipal water supply. I have my own water purification system because I need clean water to drink. Brain wellness requires chemical free, pure water so consider getting a water filter for your home or office if you think you need one. If you do not have one, you can fill up a water jug and let it stand with the lid off for several hours before drinking it. This will allow time for the gases to escape.

So, what could be more basic for supporting a healthy brain? Pack your water bottle and take frequents sips all day. There is nothing more simple or natural for you to feel better all over and keep your brain functioning. I rarely go out the door without my water bottle. You shouldn't either. **You are totally**

**in control of drinking water every day**. Make it pure. Cheers.

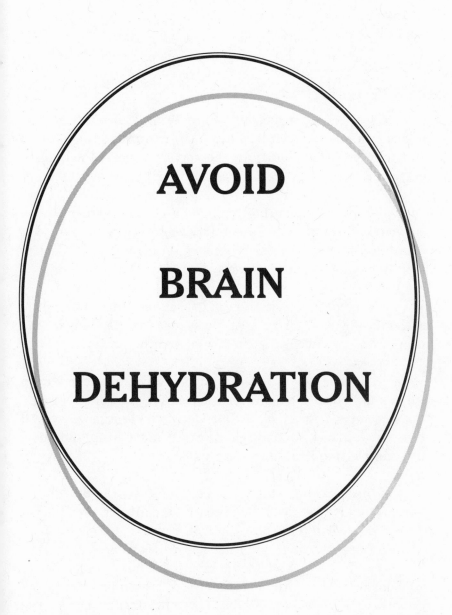

AVOID

BRAIN

DEHYDRATION

## 4.3 BREATHING

What is your breathing style? Try this little observation exercise. Lie on the floor in a comfortable position. Pay attention to your breathing. Take in a deep breath and exhale. Do this several times and observe what happened on the 'in breath'. Did your chest expand or did your abdomen expand?

**Chest Breathing**

Chest breathing is shallow breathing. It is not beneficial for your general health. Your lungs have to work hard to provide enough oxygen flow. Since only the upper portion of the lungs is being used, not enough oxygen gets into the blood system.

If you are a sloucher, you are a chest breather. If you don't sit up straight, you are restricting oxygen flow to your brain. Slouching puts a lot of tension on your muscles, not to mention having less lung capacity to use.

It's a fact that a shortage of oxygen can cause all kinds of problems. If you want to keep away drowsiness, fatigue and brain stress, you need to learn how to breathe properly.

Breathing is controlled automatically from deep within your brain. Your brain monitors the gases in your blood stream. That's good news for all of us. But, here's the best news: **we all have the ability to change our air breathing patterns anytime we need to or we want to!**

Conscious breathing can give us a tranquil mind. Consciously slowing down our breathing can turn off the constant 'monkey chatter'; those endless, repetitive thoughts that just never seem to stop. Why not learn how to breathe slower and deeper to reap the benefits of a calm mind and a better metabolism for a healthier brain? Calm breathing relaxes the sympathetic nervous system that governs stress response. The slower and deeper the rate of breathing, the deeper the thinking you can do. When your breath is fast and shallow, only superficial thinking can occur.

## Abdominal Breathing

Instead of shallow breathing, practice abdominal breathing. (Sometimes this method is called belly breathing.) Here's how.

Firstly, you should always inhale **in through your nose** and exhale **out through your nose**. This sets the pattern for calm, rhythmic breathing and the stage for self-regulation.

There are two basic tenants for abdominal breathing. The first part involves establishing a **breathing rhythm**. This is simple to do. Let's start with a two second rhythm. A second is the length of time it takes to say the words 'one thousand and one'. Begin by inhaling through your nose for the count of two seconds, hold your breath for the count of two seconds, exhale for the count of two seconds and finally, pause for the count of two seconds. This would be considered one complete breath. Practice for as long as you need to master the routine. Then you can easily extend your breathing rhythm by increasing the count to three, four, or five seconds. Build up slowly. Try at different times of the day. When you can purposely control your breathing to relax, your brain will reap the benefits.

The second part of abdominal breathing involves **inhaling deeply** into your abdomen. It is done very gently and involves no strain whatsoever. Lie on your back in a comfortable position. Place your left hand on your chest and your right hand on your belly. Inhale deeply into your abdomen so that your right hand rises. When you exhale, your right hand should drop. The left hand on your chest remains relatively still. As you take deep breaths, the right hand on your abdomen rises and falls as you inhale and exhale. This is how abdominal breathing works. It can be done lying, sitting or standing. Combine this with the self-regulation patterns above to become a competent, healthy abdominal breather.

To further enhance my life, I combine the breathing exercises with positive affirmations. For example, I repeat to myself 'breathing in I am calm, breathing out I smile' or 'breathing in I relax, breathing out I release'. Any phrase that has meaning for you is valid. It will certainly help you become more peaceful.

Luckily, we breathe all day long without thinking about it. In fact, we hardly notice it unless we run out of breath going up stairs or we get sick. With a simple conscious adjustment to our everyday breathing style, you can get healthier. Wherever you want, anytime of the day or night, you can get in touch with your breath and alter it in a positive way if you wish to. Do some research or take a course to learn more about how to breathe. **A deeper knowledge of how breathing works is one of the top secrets for brain longevity.**

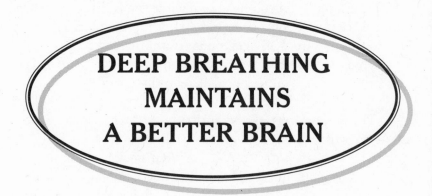

## DEEP BREATHING
## MAINTAINS
## A BETTER BRAIN

## 4.4 EXERCISE

Do you experience brain fatigue? Can't focus? Find it hard to concentrate? Feel dull and tired after sitting in front of a computer or a machine for many long hours? Worn out after caring for kids all day? BRAIN DRAIN! Everyone experiences it to a certain extent. Scientists describe these conditions as mega info-syndrome, brain bombardment or technologically induced exhaustion. These all too common conditions can be transformed even though you are tired. **Exercise** will do this for you because as soon as you start to move the brain fog will begin to lift.

The brain does not store energy. Moving your body will give you the energy you need. This is what happens in your brain when you start to move. Your whole body goes into gear. Adrenalin flows. Blood flow increases. You pay more attention. Your memory improves. Brain chemicals start to flow. Your brain circuits light up with electricity. All brain systems begin to function more efficiently creating a more balanced or homeostatic state. **YES!**

Even though your daily routine may not include an exercise program, you still may be enjoying a fully functioning brain. You may not be experiencing any sort of brain slow down or brain problems. But over time, in the long run, your brain will suffer and eventually decline if you aren't physically moving on a regular basis. You could be skipping an important daily appointment with yourself.

Have you forgotten the physical component of living? Here are some of the traditional time honoured excuses for not exercising. A person needs to buy thousands of dollars worth of home exercise equipment. The best workouts can ONLY be done at the gym. Exercise takes up too much time. There is no time to waste on exercise. I'll start next week. You have to exercise every single day to get into shape or stay in shape. Exercising hurts. Sweating is bad for you. Exercising is only for people who want big muscles or who want to look awesome in tiny bathing suits. Only young people need to exercise. Only health freaks exercise. I have this condition that stops me from doing anything. I'm resigned to living with the bulge. I'm just not into it. The list goes on and on. **Warning!** If any of these statements describe you, then you could be losing brainpower!

**It is an anatomical and physiological fact that our bodies are not meant to be stationary.** Every system in your body needs to be activated. Neuroscience is loaded with research that clearly states how absolutely necessary physical movement and aerobic exercise are for achieving optimal brain functioning and good health.

A sedentary lifestyle is an unhealthy lifestyle. Couch potatoes get a bad rep and deservedly so. What about those who must sit all day at work in front of a desk or in a vehicle? Our society is sedentary partly because we are lazy and partly because of necessity. Of greatest concern is the ever growing reality that a sedentary body means a sedentary mind. If you have to sit a lot, then there is a great need to counteract this undesirable reality. Remember, everyone is the master of his or her own brain destiny.

## A SEDENTARY LIFE IS WORSE THAN LAZY – IT'S LUNACY

In July 2004, I attended a lecture by a famous neuroscientist, Henriette Van Pragg, at the Salk Institute for Biological Studies. The Salk Institute is one of the premier brain research institutes in the world. Her talk was entitled 'Regulation of

Neurogenesis In The Adult Dentate Gyrus'. Sounds very scientific, but it was easy to understand.

Dr. Van Pragg explained that scientists are very reluctant to use the word proof. In the world of science this is what generally occurs. After years of research, a scientist publicly declares that their research findings indicate the probability of something being true by publishing it in a scientific or medical journal. Then, other scientists discuss, challenge, and copy to verify the new theory or discovery. Eventually, it is accepted as common knowledge.

The theme of this particular lecture was how aerobic exercise grows new brain cells. Dr. Van Pragg's study concluded that there was strong anatomical evidence that running produces new brain cells that are not only functional, but also superior to older ones. Her disclosures made headlines around the world. Exercise supports neurogenesis building a healthy brain and body in a host of positive ways. From her findings, an explosion of new laboratories worldwide started researching neurogenesis. Stress, aging and depression reduce neurogenesis, while movement and exercise support neurogenesis. This is why exercise infuses new life into your brain. **It is commonly accepted by scientists today that exercise grows brain cells**.

Here are some benefits of movement/exercise for your brain. Throughout thousands of years of evolution, our bodies and brains have been programmed to require movement. This holds true for anyone of any age. The brain sprouts new neurons. The brain forms newer and denser connections between neurons. Increased brain weight means more neurons and pathways have been developed.

Increased blood supply to the brain provides these benefits. Firstly, small blood vessels carrying blood can help the brain proliferate in many different places. Many brain structures can benefit from this. Exercise provides neuro protection.

The brain's structures are able to withstand brain assaults over a longer period of time improving your brain's resistance to decay. Clogging of blood vessels is lessened, which is essential to preserve brain function and reduce the risk factors for brain breakdown. Waste products, such as sticky proteins, that accumulate in the brain tissues, are carried away on a continuous basis to avoid problems.

Exercise has a positive effect on all your mental functions. There is a growing body of evidence validating the following benefits. Memory is improved. The performance of the prefrontal cortex, the executive center of your brain, also improves. Those frontal lobes are the brain's vital region for helping us make decisions in every aspect of our life. Exercise builds up your brain circuits, so that you literally have more brainpower. Your brain is more capable of blocking out endless, irrelevant stimulation. You are more able to focus and pay attention! The bottom line for us all is this – you need your mind to survive, so keep your brain alive.

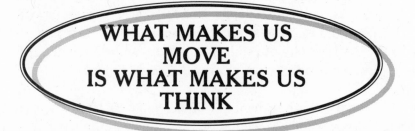

## WHAT MAKES US MOVE IS WHAT MAKES US THINK

Exercise can help you sleep better. A short walk, or a few stretches before bedtime are highly beneficial. Remember that a big time workout at the gym late at night is not a good idea as both your heart and brain can be geared up and ready to go making it hard to sleep.

Exercise is a great mood booster. Beneficial brain chemicals flood your brain, while stress hormones are eliminated. Exercise decreases anxiety and helps alleviate depression.

Exercise adds to the quality of your life! Why not boost up your feeling good neurotransmitters to beat the blues?

What is the best brain compatible exercise? **Walking.** We have bodies that are designed to walk. Walking has always been the primary form of exercise for humans. Walking can take you outside for fresh air. Walking relieves stress from tense muscles and an overworked brain. The farther and faster you walk, the more you improve the efficiency of your neural networks. Anyone can walk at any time of the day, or wherever he or she wants to. Walking is a simple exercise that is perfect for older people, younger children and everyone else. No expensive equipment is required. You don't have to be an Olympic athlete to do it. Just have a good pair of walking shoes or boots and use them regularly.

How often do you need to exercise? Naturally, this will vary greatly depending upon your lifestyle, your age and your physical condition. Exercising 4-5 times per week is what is generally recommended. Start slowly working your way up from whatever level of fitness you are at. If you have no clue nor motivation, join a class. Get some advice. There are recreation centers, gyms, and private clubs who provide fitness experts and trainers in every community. You need to stay physically fit as you age.

Don't forget that **aerobic exercise** is also needed. Sweating is healthy for you. It has direct benefits for your brain. The increased blood flow grows dendrites. It creates immediate improvements in neurological functioning. Aerobics builds both sides of your brain keeping your brain vital and alive.

This is probably the soundest advice. Do what you like to do. Do what you like to enjoy. The opportunities are endless: swim, jog, bike, climb, hike, play croquet, volleyball, basketball, indeed any sport you like. Digging in the garden is great weight training. Juggling is a super brain workout. Hackey sack, skateboarding, surfing are all wonderful activities. If you have leg or knee problems, try water workouts at the pool. Doing a variety of activities is obviously very beneficial as well as varying the routine. Consistency is the key.

Your cerebellum needs stimulation. This small structure at the back of your brain is your **balance** and co-ordination center. It needs a workout. Any activity that requires good balance is a brain enhancer. A strong cerebellum supports the prefrontal cortex and its job of problem solving, mental planning and in the co-ordination of cognitive processes. The stronger it is, the easier it is for you to think. So, exercise not only builds up your cerebellum, it literally makes you smarter.

Here's something that's fantastic for your brain. Stand on one foot. Time yourself for one or two minutes. Then, stand on the other foot. Extend your length of time to improve your balance. If this is too easy, try standing on one foot with your eyes closed. Be careful, it is not so easy to do!

Tai chi is an awesome slow motion exercise. Great flexibility and body coordination are needed to do this ancient Chinese discipline. It is well-known that yoga provides many health benefits. Dancing, skipping, tennis, racket ball, ping-pong, badminton, and golf are brain builders because they require coordinated responses to play the game. The physical activity list is endless. The secret for longevity is to exercise, increase your strength, improve your posture, balance and flexibility. This will reduce your chances of problems ahead.

The scientific data in support of exercise can't be criticized. Your biggest challenge is to get started. Make up a schedule and stick to it. Once you make a new habit it is easy to follow. After awhile, there won't be any internal debate on whether you should, or should not, do some exercise. You won't think about it, you will just do it. Exercise is the habit you want to keep your brain healthy.

# PHYSICAL FITNESS TOTALLY INFLUENCES BRAIN FITNESS

# 4.5  BRAIN GYMNASTICS ®

Brain Gymnastics® is awesome! I did brain gym in every class I taught in High School for nine years. Also, every seminar, workshop, keynote or retreat that I have the privilege of presenting at, I still do Brain Gym. These movements are very simple and easy to do. **They work!** People generally enjoy them. They bring out a lot of smiles.

About 30 years ago, it became clear that certain development movements were necessary for brain functioning. For example, a child learning to crawl at a very early age facilitates the speech and language functions of the brain. This is totally natural and part of everyone's development. Brain Gym exercises can give you the same sort of essentials at any age.

Brain Gym is a series of authentic, easy to do, fun movements. These exercises wake up your brain by activating the connections between your two hemispheres. In fact, they wake up your whole body. These movements get you ready to learn, focused, alert, clearer and stress-free. They can support you to stay centered, away from fearful brain states, or fight or flight responses. If you are having trouble doing things or thinking, try some of these on the spot movements anywhere. These exercises can improve the quality of your life and get positive changes for you **instantly**.

## Cross Overs

Benefits: the left hemisphere of your brain controls the right side of the body and the opposite is true of your right hemisphere. When you intentionally move an arm or leg across the midfield of your body, your whole brain is stimulated. Both hemispheres start working together in harmony, simultaneously.

Method: try this. With your right hand, reach over and touch your left shoulder. Drop your hand. Then with your left hand, reach over, tap your right shoulder and drop your hand. Do these shoulder taps continuously for 30 repetitions or more.

As well, try touching your elbows alternatively, then your knees. For a good challenge, lift your leg and try touching your opposite heel behind your back. Use many combinations with lots of variety. Play some uplifting music. Have fun. Get your brain unstuck. Don't forget that all movements are gentle. Physically challenged people can try doing crossovers sitting or lying down, or have someone help them. It's effortless, anyone can do it. Cross Overs are my most frequently used Brain Gym exercise.

**Brain Buttons**

Benefits: clear thinking, prepares the brain to read, stimulates brain circuits.

Method: with your thumb and index finger, make a C shape. Maintaining the C shape, place your thumb and finger on either side of your sternum just under the collarbone and massage gently the soft tissue with your fingertips. At the same time, place your other hand over your navel. Gently rub for a few seconds, change hands and repeat.

**Thinking Caps** ("Ears")

Benefits: increase the ability to hear and understand, while cutting out distracting sounds.

Method: using your thumbs, index and middle fingers, gently pull and unroll the outer part of your ears. Start from the top and gently massage to the bottom of your ears. Repeat 3 times.

**Energy Yawn**

Benefits: instant brain boost.

Method: yawning is good! It is a natural reflex your body uses to get more oxygen. Open your mouth and pretend to have a big yawn. While yawning, massage the point on your face, in front of your ears, where your upper and lower jaws meet. This brain gym exercise gets more oxygen into your brain and releases the tension in your jaw muscles. Repeat three or four times.

## Hook Ups

Benefits: defuses stress and anger, calms the emotions.

Method: cross your right ankle over your left. Extend your arms in front of you, with your thumbs pointing downwards, and cross the right wrist over the left wrist.

Interlock your fingers and draw your hands up and inwards toward your chest. Practice abdominal breathing for a minute while hooked up. Then, unlock your arms and do it again whilst crossing the left wrist over the right wrist and the left foot over the right foot.

I have used hook ups for many years to end frustration, settle arguments and disputes, returning people back to peace and harmony.

Normally, after a few minutes of anger, it takes many hours to restore balance to the immune system. Hook ups can restore balance to the immune system in 5 minutes! The fight or flight response is stopped and the frontal lobes are reawakened. Get refocused, it works!

There are several dozen Brain Gym exercises. You can't lose doing these. You can learn more about these simple coordination exercises at www.braingym.com. Try them and see if they work for you. Why live harder, when you can live smarter.

# CHAPTER 5

# Feeding Your Brain

Feeding your brain sounds odd. But, it is one of the key players you have at your disposal to keep your brain functioning well. Feeding your body to stay physically fit is a given. Feeding your brain to avoid aging and staying mentally sharp is breaking news. Nutritional strategies could be your best bet for maintaining brain health with aging. Here's some 'food for thought' for your hungry brain.

# 5.1  PROPER NUTRITION

As a brain coach, my next top strategy for you to keep your brain in shape is to be wise about nutrition. There couldn't be anything simpler in life. It is definitely one of the most important things to do for supporting your brain to function at peak levels. Isn't it logical to assume that all brains need good nutrition? Food is a powerful medium and impacts us in many ways: how we feel, how we think, the quality of our thoughts, our emotional well-being and essentially our overall health. There is a real need to be constantly watchful about what is on your plate. A top strategy to maintaining a healthy brain as well as recovering your brainpower is proper nutrition.

A healthy diet needs a good balance of proteins, fats and carbohydrates. Balanced meals mean balanced minds. There are lots of diets on the market. If you want to change or improve your diet, seek the expert advice of a health care professional. The key is to become educated.

**Proteins** give you stamina, balance your blood-sugar levels and manufacture neurotransmitters. Protein is an essential component of your neurons. No protein, no brain growth. Good sources are nuts, seeds, nut butters, eggs, beans, fish and white meats.

**Carbohydrates** provide energy and stress reduction. Simple carbohydrates (white bread, donuts, white flour, etc.) are not recommended. Complex carbohydrates (100% whole wheat, whole grains, fruits and vegetables) are recommended. Foods like whole wheat bread and brown rice allow for slower digestion, a gradual rise in blood sugar and a gradual lowering of blood sugar.

If your work is entirely mental, then eat more proteins. After a meal of mainly protein, you will be able to stay more focused. So, if you want a sharp brain all day, have protein at every meal. Have light carbohydrates for lunch and save the potatoes and pasta for dinner. Bottom line: If you want to relax after a meal, eat carbohydrates. If you want to be mentally alert, eat protein.

Breakfast is the most important meal of the day. Your seven-and-a-half hours of sleep means seven-and-a-half hours of fasting. Breakfast is breaking the fast. Neurons cannot store glucose as they readily use it up. Therefore, glucose is needed for your brain to function if you want to have a great day. A combination of foods that provide a slow and sustained energy source is ideal. A superior breakfast would be:

## fruit or fruit juice + protein + whole grain

Most nutrition experts recommend eating three balanced meals a day. Going over four to five hours without a meal is too draining. The brain benefits from small snacks between meals so that there is a constant supply of glucose. Some great choices for snacks are trail mixes, cut up vegetables, fresh fruits, pita bread and hummus, yogurt, smoothies, or protein drinks. Make good snack choices because they have a direct impact on your quality of life.

Neurotransmitters are the messenger carriers in your brain. Thinking and learning are biochemical processes that require these chemicals. Here are some of the brain foods you need to have in your diet to produce them.

**Acetylcholine** – for memory support. Eat foods with choline in them such as egg yolks, nuts, wheat germ and cauliflower. Also eat foods that contain lecithin such as peanuts, soybeans, or wheat germ.

**Serotonin** – to stay calm, concentrated and relaxed. Eat complex carbohydrates such as whole grain cereals, whole wheat breads, brown rice, pasta, potatoes and starchy vegetables.

**Dopamine** – to stay alert, focused and energized. Eat protein foods such as beans, nuts, fish, turkey and soy products.

## MAKE SURE YOUR BRAIN IS NOT MALNOURISHED

## 5.2 FABULOUS FISH

Your brain needs a special **fat** called Omega 3. The neurons in your brain are rich in Omega 3 and brain cells cannot function without it. This fat is needed to grow dendrites and synapses so that they can send messages throughout your brain.

Omega 3 is made up of two fatty acids that are the big players in your brain chemistry. The first one is called **DHA** (docosahexaenoic acid). DHA is the very best brain fat. It has been shown to enhance memory, attention span, intelligence and overall mental functioning. DHA is used to manage attention deficit disorder and other learning disabilities. DHA supplements are of support to people with dementia and memory loss. If you want to improve your brain health, make sure DHA is in your diet.

The second fatty acid is called **EPA** (eicosapentaenoic acid). It is significant for keeping your moods stable. Feeling good requires EPA in your brain to alleviate anxiety or depression. It is therefore of great significance for you to have DHA and EPA in your diet to keep your brain vital and alive. Omega 3 supplies them.

The best sources of Omega 3 are fish. Since the body cannot make these essential fats, they have to be obtained through food. At the top of the recommended list is salmon, *wild sockeye salmon*. Sockeye salmon is loaded with high levels of Omega 3. Wild British Columbia salmon harvested in the Pacific Ocean ranks at the top of the brain food list. It is a delicious and superior food source.

If you are concerned about toxins, like mercury, check out Canada's seafood guide at www.seachoice.org. It is a good place for you to find out your best choices. Fish are rated under three categories: best choice, some concerns, and avoid. Make informed intelligent choices, especially when it comes to the super star brain food. Other recommended fish species are: lake trout, tuna, sole, snapper and cod. A good policy is to eat fish twice a week.

In addition to eating fish, I take purified fish oils daily. Triple fish oils are excellent. They contain sardines, mackerel and anchovies, which are cold, deep-water fish that come from the shores of South America. Triple fish oils are rich in EPA and DHA. These oils are safer and cleaner than fish itself. Manufacturers who make purified oils claim that they are toxic free.

When I was a child, every morning for years and years my mother would give me a spoonful of cod liver oil. Today, I am still taking that spoonful of cod liver oil. Our parents, grandparents and great grandparents knew that fish was brain food. They didn't need scientists or experts to tell them. They were right.

If you have a good brain and want to keep it that way, then take Omega 3 every day. If you want to regenerate your brain, then you have to have Omega 3 to get you there. Your brain grows, changes, shapes, prunes, reshapes, rewires, and reconnects constantly. If you want to totally support your brain's natural activities, Omega 3 is the answer.

Other OMEGA 3 sources:

I eat a lot of organic flax seeds. Every morning I grind them up for breakfast. I prefer them this way, rather than taking flax seed oil, because they are always fresh. Eggs are an excellent source of omega 3 oils. Walnuts, pumpkin seeds, olive oil, peanut butter, avocadoes, and hemp seeds are also excellent sources.

# SMART
# BRAIN OWNERS
# EAT OMEGA 3
# RICH FOODS

# 5.3 ANTIOXIDANTS Vs FREE RADICALS

There are battles going on in your brain, especially if you are experiencing signs of brain aging. An enemy is draining your brainpower, erasing your memory and fogging your brain. It is the source of many brain problems including degenerative diseases. These antagonists are called **free radicals**.

Your brain is a very active organ. Twenty percent of your total oxygen intake is consumed by your three pound brain. It takes glucose and oxygen to make energy. So every time your brain makes energy, billions of neurons burn white hot. Unfortunately, oxygen molecules break loose becoming those toxic substances called free radicals.

Free radicals are unstable and they like to bond with other molecules in healthy cells. This bonding process causes heat. Heat damages the cell membranes of your neurons. This action is called **oxidation** (oxidative stress). Destruction to your brain cells is the result. These unstable free radicals are your enemy. They are bullies who constantly attack and kill brain cells.

A second major dilemma literally gives you headaches. The energy producing centers of your brain cells are called MITOCHONDRIA. Free radicals disrupt the production of energy in the brain cells and destroy these mitochondria. Less energy is produced and efficiency is lost. It's a vicious cycle. Free radicals are zapping your brain strength. It gets harder to concentrate. You get fatigued more easily. You are more vulnerable to stress, thus supporting the production of more free radicals.

A third problem is that these free radicals disrupt the production of neurotransmitters. Thus communication between brain cells is less efficient, which negatively impacts all your cognitive functions. Free radicals are working in your brain as you read this book. Every second, every minute, every day of your life, free radicals attack.

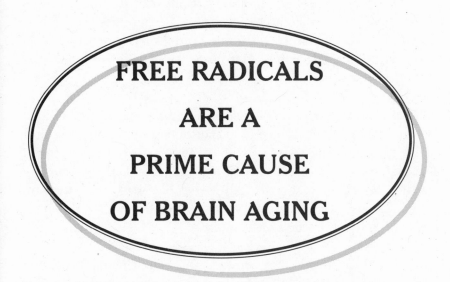

FREE RADICALS
ARE A
PRIME CAUSE
OF BRAIN AGING

Maintaining a healthy youthful brain depends upon your ability to combat free radical production. In order to do this, you need **antioxidants** to win the brain war.

Antioxidants to the rescue! Mother Nature knows best. Your body has already got a built-in defense system in place. Free radical attack and damage need to be kept in check. The oxidation process continues constantly. Fortunately, so does the antioxidant protection plan. Antioxidants catch and wipe out the free radicals stopping free radical damage. **Yes!** Some antioxidants are produced in the body, while others have to be obtained from your diet. The battle between free radicals and antioxidants is literally at the core of aging. The wrinkles on your face, the graying of your hair, the dimming of your eyes, the gradual slowing down of your body and its health related problems are all about which of these two players are winning the oxidation battle.

**Eat vegetables**. There are many naturally occurring

food sources that can provide you with the antioxidants you need to slow down your mental and physical decline. Start by eating colourful vegetables everyday. Vegetables are full of antioxidants, including vitamins and healthy **polyphenols** (powerful micronutrients)! Many scientists believe that vegetables increase antioxidant activity.

It is possible now for scientists to analyze how quickly antioxidants in vegetables (and fruits) can eliminate free radicals. Here are the top antioxidant super stars: kale, spinach, brussel sprouts, broccoli, beets, onions, peas, cabbage, carrots, beans, celery and squash. All vegetables are good for you. Vegetables are friendly foods that supply fibre, water, minerals, and those much needed antioxidants.

**Eat fruits**. Fruits are also full of antioxidants. People who eat a lot of fruit daily reduce the risk of developing disease. Eat fruit that is fresh and in season. Prunes and plums are some of the best to eat. Eat tomatoes. They are a fine source of **lycopene** – a superior antioxidant. An apple a day keeps the doctor away is the old saying. This is true because apples are a very rich source of antioxidants.

Other healthy antioxidant fruits are: avocados, grapes, bananas, cherries, grapefruits, watermelon, nectarines, oranges, peaches, pears, and pineapples.

Which food source in the world provides the most antioxidant protection? **Blueberries!** Research reported in Scientific Journals around the world continually confirms the wide range of health benefits provided by blueberries. Over and over again, research laboratories are saying: blueberries are brain berries. Why? Blueberries have the highest antioxidant capacity of all fruits and vegetables. They fight inflammation. Blackberries, strawberries, and raspberries are also recommended.

**Eat Organic Foods**. Certified organic means that you

are eating pesticide free, chemical free products. It's a no-brainer to see that you get more value from organic produce in terms of vitamins and minerals than produce from denatured, denurtured commercial products. Yes, it does cost more but aren't you and your family worth it? Support your local organic producers. They are important for our future as a healthy society.

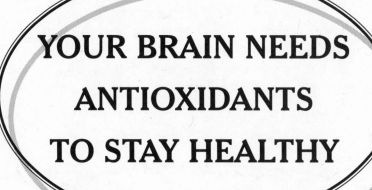

YOUR BRAIN NEEDS
ANTIOXIDANTS
TO STAY HEALTHY

## 5.4 RESTRICT THOSE CALORIES

The researchers of today are saying very clearly "eat less and live longer". Yet, so many people are eating themselves to death. The current epidemic of obesity will soon become the epidemic of brain degeneration. Obesity often causes fading mental faculties. Not only does packing on the pounds put a strain on your heart, it can also age your brain faster. Unrestricted eating accelerates brain aging. Find out what portion size is right for you and stick to it.

**Excessive calories damage neurons**. Here's how. When you process calories by metabolizing them, oxygen must be burned. As you know, this process creates free radicals that damage neurons. Every calorie you eat must be burned. Excess calories mean more free radical damage because the more you eat the more oxygen has to be burned to process them. Thus, calorie restriction slows down aging not only throughout your whole body, but particularly your brain. Eating a lighter diet, without starving, will support brain longevity.

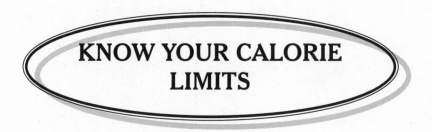

KNOW YOUR CALORIE
LIMITS

# 5.5 BRAIN BUILDING FOODS

**Whole Grains**: oatmeal is one of the best foods for your brain. Oats are a carbohydrate rich food that will supply you with a shot of glucose to jump start your brain. The higher the concentration of glucose in your blood, the better your memory and brainpower will be.

We all need to eat more whole grains such as barley, rye, whole wheat and wheat bran. They are rich in fibre. They are also rich in antioxidants and **lignans**. Lignans are wonderful protective substances that are getting a lot of attention lately.

Read the package. Avoid products whose ingredients state: enriched, goodness of enriched or added fibre. These are all refined products that are not as good as intact fibre. Go for the natural grains!

**Seeds And Nuts**: here are some great choices that are best eaten raw and unsalted. Brazil nuts contain selenium, which provide antioxidant protection. Almonds are rich in vitamin E. Have you noticed that walnuts look like a brain? Walnuts are an excellent source of Omega 3. Sprouts (alfalfa, radish, sunflower, mung beans) are great for salads, sandwiches and roll ups. My refrigerator always contains almond butter, cashew butter, tahini butter (sesame seeds) and hemp seed nut butter. Go nuts!

**Herbs**: don't forget these. Herbs are powerful free radical suppressors. Herbs, often dried, are used to flavour foods or for medicinal purposes. Cook with some of these fresh as often as you can: rosemary, dill, sage, mint, basil, garlic, thyme, parsley, and coriander are only a few to choose from. Sprinkle them on your salads, vegetables, and cook them in your soups. They add flavour, aroma and aid digestion. Ayurvedic medicine, the oldest traditional medicine in India, highly recommends herbs to build your brainpower. Furthermore, make sure your kitchen cabinet has several salt free herbal mix seasonings to choose from.

**Spices**: spices also contain antioxidants. Lots of our favourite foods from around the world contain spices. Here are just a few: black pepper, cardamon, cloves, ginger, nutmeg, cinnamon. They enhance our foods making them super delicious. Of special note are ginger and turmeric because they are antioxidants and have anti-inflammatory benefits. Curcumin is currently very highly recommended. It is the yellow pigment in turmeric. Curcumin is being used to treat Alzheimer's disease. Finally, it's good for us all to limit our intake of salt. If you use salt, then natural sea salt, free of additives and preservatives, is nature's best product.

**Good Fat**: as you know fat is necessary in our diet because brain cells contain fat. Moderation of course is the key. Good healthy sources are available from avocados, nuts and fish. These are good choices to support mental clarity and concentration. The right fats are fabulous!

**Oils**: olive oil is a top choice. It is a very stable oil that does not need refrigeration. Buy cold pressed extra-virgin organic olive oil. It's good for your brain and your skin. Other choices include: hemp oil, sesame oil, grape seed oil, walnut oil, soybean oil and pumpkin seed oil. Also, don't forget those daily fish oils.

**Legumes**: legumes are an excellent meat alternative supplying protein. Legumes are high in B vitamins and low in saturated fat. For a balanced meal, combine them with brown rice or whole wheat pasta. Good choices are beans, peas, lentils or tofu. Look ahead to getting more protein from plant sources.

**Poultry**: choose white meat for your diet. Make it free-range organic chicken or turkey.

**Meat**: lean meat is the best choice. It's no secret that too much saturated fat is not good for us.

**Drinks**: the top drink for your brain is pure water. Add a slice of lemon or lime to give a hint of flavour. You can also enjoy herbal non-caffeinated teas, vegetable juices and fruit juices.

**Green Tea**: in recent years, green tea has risen to the heights of recommended brain nutrients. Green tea has beneficial nutrients, polyphenols, which provide antioxidant protection. Green tea is a superstar brain food.

**Snacks**: if you want to be at your personal brain best, consider this question whenever you get a hunger attack. Will this snack keep my brain healthy or will this snack accelerate its aging?

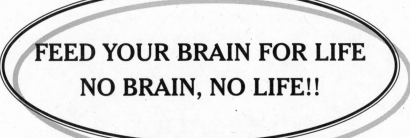

FEED YOUR BRAIN FOR LIFE
NO BRAIN, NO LIFE!!

## 5.6 VITAMINS AND MINERALS

Do we need to take supplements? **Definitely yes!** Supplements do not replace a good diet, but they can help avoid nutrient deficiencies. There are still people around who argue that you can get all the nutrients you need from a normal diet. Not any more. The food supply is depleted by modern food processing methods. The commercial food supply is not nutritionally adequate.

Perhaps the biggest compelling argument in favour of supplements is the lifestyle of the average Canadian. If you are not eating a balanced diet, it will take its toll on your brain. Supplements are needed because we are not mindful enough about our diets. So often our way of living does not support health and wellness. These neuro-nutrients are needed to make your brain strong protecting you from dementia.

If a few supplements a day support your brain health, reduce the risk of future brain problems and keep brain disease at bay, isn't this one of the best investments that you can make?

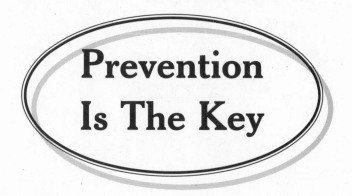

**Prevention Is The Key**

### Vitamins

Seek advice from qualified people. I get my vitamins from a Health Food Store and my Naturopathic Doctor. Buy vitamins that have no sugar, no starch, no artificial colours, no artificial flavours and no preservatives. Remember that risk factors are low.

Vitamins can do many things for your brain. The evidence is totally compelling. Vitamins protect young healthy brains and stave off intellectual deterioration over time, especially for anyone over the age of 30. If you are a baby-boomer who has eaten a lousy diet for decades, you may need vitamin support. You can't see what is going on in your brain but if you get sick, your brain has probably been impoverished or suffering long before the physical signs show up. Why not do what you can to avoid problems in the first place? Research concludes that older people with high blood levels of vitamins are farther ahead of everyone else their age! Vitamins are anti-senility nutrients. The overall message is take vitamins to maintain your brain faculties for a whole lifetime regardless of your age.

## The Vitamin B Complex

The B vitamins are essential to support the growth of neurons and for keeping your brain alive and well. Taking a basic B complex supplement is a wise thing to do. B's are especially effective to counteract stress. They support a healthy nervous system. Most importantly, they are needed to synthesize neurotransmitters to support your mood and your thinking. B vitamins need to be taken daily because they are water-soluble and can be excreted from the body.

Seniors especially need to be aware of vitamin deficiencies. Their diets often get restricted because they tend to eat the same foods all the time. Seniors need B vitamins as much as anyone. The B's are critical to preserving aging brains, keeping away depression and preventing dementia. Since subtle deficiencies inside the brain cannot be seen, why take a chance? B complex vitamins are found in a wide variety of products including: whole grain cereals, eggs, nuts, fish, fruits and green vegetables.

## Vitamin B12

This vitamin is very important. Vitamin B12 produces and maintains myelin in the brain. Myelin is the protective covering around the axon of your neurons. Unfortunately, myelin breaks down during aging. Brain cells can be damaged compromising memory and slowing down your thinking. Loss of myelin is a major reason why the brain shrinks. Vitamin B12 is mainly supplied from meat in your diet. Vegetarians can get B12 from eggs, fish and dairy products.

## Vitamin C

Your body cannot make its own vitamin C. It has to come from your diet or from supplements. **Vitamin C is absolutely critical for your brain.** Your brain needs more vitamin C than any other part of your body. Your brain literally doesn't function well without it. What does it do for your brain? It is an essential ingredient for creating the neurotransmitters – acetylcholine and dopamine. It therefore plays a major role in brain biochemistry. Next, vitamin C is a super antioxidant. It is present in the fluid around neurons protecting them from free radical attack. As well, vitamin C helps boost the effectiveness of vitamin E, another important antioxidant. Obviously, it is very important to have a good supply in your body everyday. It is safe to take, according to most sources, and easy to obtain. Vitamin C is a superstar brain booster and brain preserver. Fruits like oranges and grapefruits are rich in this vitamin.

## Vitamin D

Vitamin D is a hot topic today. Many Canadians are deficient almost all year round because we do not get enough sunlight. Vitamin D is essential for maintaining a positive mood. It also provides antioxidant protection from free radical attack. If you are concerned about brain aging and your overall health, Vitamin D may help reduce your risks.

### Vitamin E

Scientists call vitamin E **The Smart Pill**. In all of nature, it is one of the most powerful antioxidants known to exist. Vitamin E protects cell membranes from free radical attack. It guards, protects and preserves what you need to have – brain cells. There is a **ton** of scientific evidence supporting the efficacy of vitamin E to help you reduce the risk of not only brain diseases but other diseases as well. Vitamin C and vitamin E need to be taken together. Oils, nuts and seeds are natural sources.

### Minerals

It would be very wise to take trace minerals. Many multivitamin formulas contain minerals for a good reason. Minerals are a part of the nutrient rich diet needed to keep your aging brain cells healthy and vital. People who are experiencing cognitive decline are often deficient in minerals. For example, your brain needs magnesium to function as well as helping to slow down the aging process. Minerals act as catalysts to allow vitamins to do their job. I take sea minerals daily. I take ten to twelve drops in a small glass of water. It tastes terrible but it is good medicine.

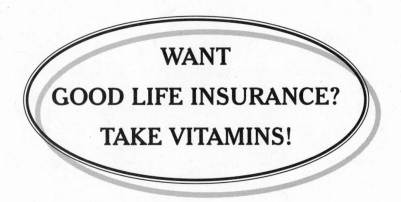

WANT
GOOD LIFE INSURANCE?
TAKE VITAMINS!

## 5.7  THE SUPER BRAIN BOOSTERS

These exquisite natural supplements can support you to improve normal brain function. They also can support you to prevent disease and illness. These brain supplements are major players in any intelligent brain longevity program. They are some of the most potent brain protective nutrients available today.

### Lecithin

Your brain cells are made of a natural substance called lecithin. It is a key structural material for the brain. Why? Lecithin is needed to build a strong network of neurons with trillions of connections between them. Taking lots of lecithin in your diet delays brain aging and, therefore, could improve your mental function. It's a brain protector. As well, lecithin is needed to produce acetylcholine, the neurotransmitter responsible for memory and thinking. Regardless of age, everyone needs lecithin in their diet to keep their memory systems working and to build the myelin sheath surrounding the axon. Your body cannot make enough of it for you. Without it you cannot store memories. Don't forget, myelin loss could mean memory loss. Your brain will not function properly unless you have lecithin in your diet.

Lecithin is readily available from health food stores. It does not cure brain problems but acts as a beneficial, preventative agent. It is not expensive and no prescription is needed to purchase it. There are no known side effects. I have taken lecithin in granular form for over 20 years. My wife takes her daily lecithin in glycerin capsules. It's definitely a super brain booster. The best food sources are soya beans, egg yolks, peas, beans, tofu products and green leafy vegetables.

### Ginkgo Biloba

Ginkgo Biloba is an awesome natural remedy. Ginkgo

has been used by the Chinese for thousands of years as a general brain tonic. It is one of the most extensively studied plant supplements. Hundreds of studies (scientifically controlled, double-blind experiments) have demonstrated that ginkgo improves mental functioning. Ginkgo's most valuable assets are: it increases blood flow to the brain, it increases oxygen to the brain, it improves memory and it increases mental alertness. Ginkgo is slow acting. You probably won't get your memory back overnight if that's what you expect. Ginkgo is not a cure all for dementia or other diseases, but it is of value for delaying cognitive decline as we age. Be sure to buy ginkgo with at least 24% concentration of the active ingredient. If you have memory problems or are at risk for memory problems, consider Ginkgo Biloba.

## Phosphatidylserine

Phosphatidylserine, commonly known as PS, is a super star brain tonic. PS is a fat that is found in all your body cells, not just your brain cells. We manufacture it naturally but its production in the body declines with age. It keeps the cell membranes permeable so that nutrients can enter the cell and wastes can leave. Thus, PS is absolutely indispensable for healthy cell membranes. Brain cells need it to communicate easily with each other. If you are always misplacing things or can't remember the name of something, your cells are not communicating very well. There is great hope that this nutrient can help people avoid memory impairment because it boosts acetylcholine.

## Co-Enzyme Q-10

Your body produces Co-Enzyme Q-10 naturally. Co-Enzyme Q-10 is absolutely vital for brain health as it helps support energy production in the brain cells. The brain cannot perform all of its essential tasks without it. If the brain is short of fuel it cannot think, learn or remember. Without Co-Enzyme Q-10, your brain won't work and if you do not produce enough of it, your brain will degenerate faster. As well, it is an antioxidant and provides protection against free radicals. It is critical for maintaining brain longevity. A great concern is the fact that, unfortunately, production of it in your body declines with age and that is why it is so very highly recommended by neuroscientists. If you are low on energy and experience brain fatigue, then Co-Enzyme Q-10 may be of help to you.

## Ginseng

Another herb from the Orient, Ginseng has positive neurological effects on the brain. It has been used in Asia since antiquity. It's greatest value is in its ability to act as an ADAPTOGEN – a substance that helps the body counteract many types of stress, both physical and mental. Ginseng moderates stress that can decrease your mental performance. Therefore, it promotes clear thinking and gives you mental stamina. The greatest benefit is its strength at stopping the production of CORTISOL (see Brain Killers 6.1). Researchers have documented ginseng's ability to improve the mental performance of people who have to live and work under constant stress, as well as improve the mental performance of healthy people. There are many types and brands of ginseng. Do your research and experiment to find the one that best suits your needs.

## Green Drinks

My day starts with a green drink. Here are some of the wonderful life enhancing ingredients in my green drink: bee pollen, dulse, green tea, licorice root, ginkgo, milk thistle, chlorella, barley grass, wheat grass and many more, **all** of which are natural brain tonics. With every glass, I get a wide variety of micronutrients that I can't get in most common foods!

**Chlorella**, for example, is nutritious green algae. It is the most popular food supplement in Japan. It contains essential amino acids that the body can't manufacture on its own. No amino acids, no neurotransmitters.

Green juices made from barley or wheat grass have been popular for decades. No wonder! It is recommended to have your green drink first thing in the morning. It will get your brainpower started naturally for the day. Better than coffee!

A final comment about feeding your brain is necessary. Skillful use of nutrition and nutritional supplements will supply you with the brainpower you need. These brain builders come from Mother Nature. They build a strong organic core for your brain. You can't think unless you have good chemistry. That means putting live food into your body to make neurotransmitters. You don't have any memory without myelin so get lecithin into your diet and your children's diet. You haven't any brain cells without the essential Omega 3s. Since we are exposed to rising toxicity from our polluted environment, we eat chemically loaded, processed foods. We eat on the run, skip meals, and we forget to feed our brain. Why wait for a brain breakdown, or a stroke, or Alzheimer's disease? Spend a little time and effort to avoid problems and enjoy your brain as you age.

There is a common occurrence in my Brain Wellness presentations. Invariably someone will ask the big question which usually sounds like this "Why do we have to take all this stuff?" I always answer with the truth. **"To avoid brain rot!"**

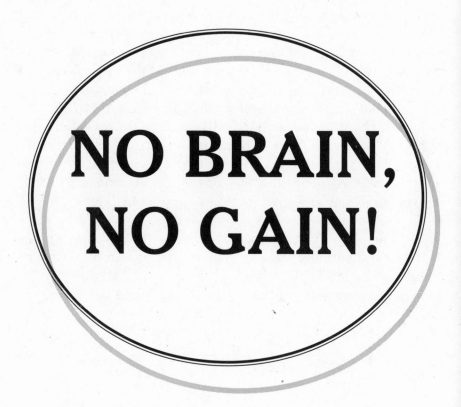

NO BRAIN,
NO GAIN!

# 6
# Chapter

# Brain Killers

Neuroscientists are sounding the alarm bells. Canadian baby boomers are facing a tidal wave of dementia. This mind destroying epidemic will decimate tens of thousands of baby boomers who will soon be retiring. The golden years won't be so golden. The following brain killers all contribute to the ultimate tragedy feared by so many aging people.

# 6.1 CORTISOL & THE STRESSED OUT BRAIN

Are you living with a stressed out brain? Many people do. They live and work in a stressful environment and are not even aware of it. They don't know that their brain is under stress because that's the way they live. It's hard to escape. There is too much to do, too much going on. The pressure of living just never ends. We all experience both acute and chronic levels of stress at different times of our life. Life was easier before, but today the stressers of modern life are increasing dramatically. The rat race will continue to accelerate. More synapses will sizzle. Trying to get rid of stress is an illusion for many of us. Stress elimination can be a challenge. So, what's the answer? **Stress management!**

The constant stimulation on our nervous system is relentless. Cell phones, emails, television commercials, machines, noise, appointments, and deadlines are just a few of the endless lineup of experiences in today's world. Stress can be exciting and uplifting like starting a new job, a new relationship, or travel. But, on the flip side, if you experience a lot of headaches, backaches, poor digestion problems, bite your nails, worry a lot, have a short fuse or are irritable, and just feel over extended, then that's an indication of too much stress. **Excess stress destroys your brainpower**.

When you are under real or imaginary stress your body reacts. Two major hormones are produced which pour into your body. **Adrenalin** and **cortisol** are released by the adrenal glands located just above your kidneys. Blood flow goes to your arms and legs. Your breathing rate and your heart rate increase. Your muscles are ready to work. These two hormones get you out of trouble. They are the primary chemicals of the **Fight or Flight** response. Under ideal conditions, adrenalin and cortisol eventually shut off and their effects dissipate.

We forget that our brain is flesh and blood. We need to be aware of how the stress response in your body operates. The fight or flight response is an essential tool for your survival. It's fantastic and you need it. It developed very early in our evolution when most of our threats were physical. When you were threatened, you ran away. Today's threats are very different. They do not require a physical response because the threats are mental or emotional rather than physical. But, non-physical stress creates the same reaction with the production of adrenalin and cortisol.

The Cortisol Connection:

*"Cortisol is one of the hormones secreted by the adrenal glands. It's secreted in response to stress. In moderate amounts, cortisol is not harmful. But when produced in excess, day after day – as a result of chronic, unrelenting stress – this hormone is so toxic to the brain that it kills and injures brain cells by the billions."*
Dr. Dharma Singh Khalsa, M.D.
*Brain Longevity*

Cortisol goes into the hippocampus of your brain. That's one way your **memory** is being destroyed. The more stress you have, the more cortisol you produce. Your chances of developing memory loss increase. Too much cortisol is like pouring battery acid into your brain. Your hippocampus gets a toxic bath. Cells die. The telephone lines go down. Communication is disrupted. Sometimes your mind goes blank. Sometimes you get a little confused when the pressure is on. Many of us have experienced these signs but don't recognize the underlying dangers. Because of chronic stress your hippocampus gradually begins to shrink and atrophy. The cycle of degeneration is on, full speed ahead. Alzheimer sufferers have higher levels of cortisol than normal aging people. Cortisol is an acclaimed brain killer.

The solution is that you have to learn how to cut off the

chronic stress response buttons because stress is eating away your vital brainpower. Premature brain aging is a serious issue. The relationship between chronic stress and mental decline is unmistakable. Don't be a passive young adult or an aging baby boomer. Find out how to handle your stress. Why wait for the melt down?

**TOO MUCH CORTISOL
PREVENTS
YOUR BRAIN FROM
LAYING DOWN
MEMORY**

# 6.2  SLEEP DEPRIVATION

Who isn't living a busy life these days? For too many of us, sleep is something you squeeze in between everything else you have to do. But, the reality is that your brain is only good for 16 hours a day. After that, it can't function as efficiently.

All humans have a natural sleep clock. Our bodies work on 24-hour cycles called **Circadian Rhythms**. The word circadian means 'about one day'. These rhythms control our sleep/wake cycles.

Signals are constantly being sent to the brain from the eyes. When it gets dark, the brain starts to secret Melatonin. This hormone is what puts us to sleep. When morning light hits the eyes, a message is sent to the brain to be more attentive. It's time to wake up. Melatonin production stops. Thus, exposure to sunlight determines when we need to be awake and when we need to sleep.

If you stay up late at night, are you really getting ahead? Or are you depriving yourself of something that is essential for your wellbeing? Today's adults need between seven to nine hours sleep a night to feel their best. Adolescents and children need more.

One hundred years ago, most Canadians averaged 9 to 9½ hours of sleep per night. That was before light bulbs and other inventions became available to everyone. Lights have extended our days and increased the wear and tear on our brains.

If you are getting less than seven hours a night, you may be **sleep deprived**. It is one of the main causes of so much of the fatigue and exhaustion that contributes to a problematic **sleep debt**. Unfortunately, sleep debt becomes a way of life. People don't notice how tired they are. We have adapted to new levels of permanent drowsiness. If we are getting an hour less each night of what we need, that's a lot of hours by the end of the year in our fast paced 24/7 world. Are you getting adequate amounts of sleep?

What goes on in your brain if you don't get enough sleep? Lots! Lack of sleep eats away at your brain cells. Every night your brain needs time to repair its cells. It also makes new ones. The neurons slow down their activity to clean out wastes. Also, sleep allows the levels of neurotransmitters to be normalized. Without rest, the lack of sleep actually promotes free radical production.

**Memories form at night**. A good sleep makes a big difference about how we can remember. Connections between neurons are strengthened to support memory. The brain sorts, rearranges and literally dumps useless information during sleep. It stores what it regards as important. Circuits need time to do this housekeeping work. If not enough sleep is obtained, storage and repair work can't get done and we forget more easily. We won't get optimal brain performance the next day and our memory won't be as sharp.

What can happen to **you** when you don't get enough sleep? Sleep is a time when most body systems shut down and rest. The heart rate lowers, blood pressure lowers as well as your overall metabolism. As we all know, lack of sleep affects our cognitive and physical functions. Our defense cells are weakened which makes us more vulnerable to infections and diseases. Our bodies are under stress and they pump out more stress hormones. If you do not charge up your batteries, they can't provide you with much power. Lack of sleep decreases your ability to think clearly. Lack of sleep affects your ability to pay attention, make good judgments or solve problems. It can put you into a negative mood, decrease your productivity and increase chances for errors. A good sleep makes a HUGE difference to how we function on a day-to-day basis.

In conclusion, it is critical for the brain to be rested.

There are a whole host of benefits. Sleep impairment is becoming a most common brain impairment for people of all ages. If you want to be mentally sharp, then get a good night's sleep. The brain is the key organ in your body; give it what it needs.

**Over time sleep deprivation will destroy the integrity of your brain**

## 6.3 BRAIN INFLAMMATION

Your body's first line of defense against unwanted invaders is inflammation. It's the body's natural reaction against threats. When you cut your finger, it swells up. If you bash your elbow, it swells up. That's the age-old immunological system at work. It's designed to be your lifesaver. This process is critical for maintaining your health **unless** the inflammatory process becomes chronic. Then, your protection mechanism no longer switches off. Trouble!

How could inflammation possibly get into your brain? Easy. The stimulus that triggers it occurs when you eat a diet of high sugar, trans fatty acids, smoke cigarettes, drink alcohol, don't exercise, don't get enough sleep, live with too much stress, or generally neglect your health. Millions of people trigger inflammation in their brain in these ways and are totally unaware of the damage they are doing to themselves.

Inflammation is hard to see. It's silent. Free radicals promote inflammation. The immune system attacks threatening invaders automatically. This can create more free radicals, which in turn can create more inflammation. Inflammation damage spreads to neighbouring cells triggering more inflammation. An accelerating spiral of decline continues day after day. The **off switch** no longer works wreaking havoc on your neurons. The destruction becomes self-perpetuating.

Inflammation is one of the hottest areas of research in the world today. Alzheimer's and other brain diseases are characterized by classic inflammation of neural tissues. Preventative steps are needed which would include eating anti-inflammatory foods in your diet, taking supplements, exercising and getting lots of sleep. Make sure your body's inflammatory switch is turned "on" only when it needs to be.

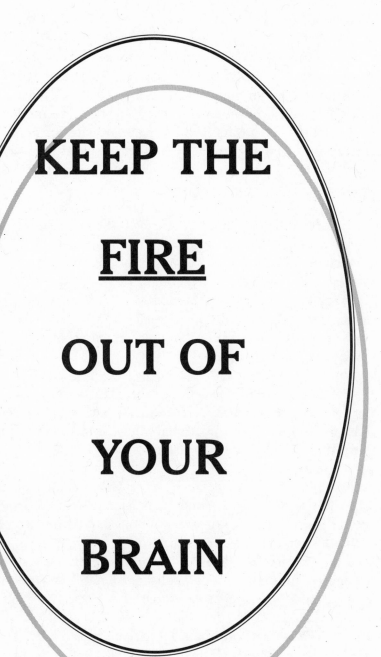

KEEP THE

<u>FIRE</u>

OUT OF

YOUR

BRAIN

# 6.4 JUNK FOOD

Junk food is a very common term that has been around for many years. It describes food that has no nutritional value or is unhealthy for you. What's wrong with it? Typically it contains high levels of salt, sugar, fat, food additives and lacks vitamins, fibre, and proteins. It is popular with so many people because it's easy to purchase and it tastes good. Over consumption of undesirable junk food is directly related to many diseases.

Junk food is empty caloric food. It has energy content but lacks vitamins and minerals. On the market today, there are thousands and thousands of junk food products. An occasional order of fries won't kill you. But if this is your regular fare: a breakfast of coffee and doughnuts; a lunch of fries, packaged snacks with pop; and finally, a greasy fast food supper, look out. You need **diet reform**. I highly recommend that you watch the movie "Super Size Me".

Obviously this is a huge topic. The bottom line is, what you eat will immediately have a huge effect on your brain today and tomorrow. Poor nutritional choices are often behind our current epidemic of poor brain functioning.

**Fat.** Some fats are good, some aren't. **Monosaturated** fat from olive oil, sesame oil, almond oil is good. **Saturated** fat is not good. The messages are everywhere. Cut down on your consumption of animal products to support your own personal health. Eating less meat fights climate change, supports a cleaner environment and a healthier planet. You can easily get your protein from vegetable sources.

**Trans fatty acids** are a serious health risk. These are chemicals created by Industry. They do not exist in Nature. They are 100% synthetic. Chemicals like hydrogenated oils and margarine are trans fatty acids. They are added to foods to extend shelf life. Baked goods and fried foods contain them. I will always remember a documentary on the Nature Of Things with David Suzuki. Margarine and butter were being compared. Time and time again, rodents were offered these two as food. The rodents would always eat the butter. The rodents never ate the margarine. In December 2006, the city of New York banned all trans fatty acids from food sold in restaurants. That's a huge paradigm shift in favour of protecting the general public. More and more products have a 'no trans fat' notice on the packaging. YES! These bad fats make your brain cells rigid. Nutrients can't get in while wastes can't get out, inviting free radicals to destroy your cells. If you value your brain health, follow these positive trends. Check your cupboards and throw away anything with trans fatty acids in them. Avoid the nightmares. Eliminate the bad fat. Increase the good fat.

**Sugar.** "White death" or white table sugar has huge adverse effects on the body. It is grown in fields with chemicals, cooked, processed and stripped of any nutritional value. No living organisms are left in it. Once in Queensland, Australia, I stood in one of the biggest buildings I have ever been in. It was full of mountains of brown cane sugar. The smell was overpowering. It was hard to breathe. Bulldozers were pushing the sugar onto conveyor belts, which emptied into a bulk tanker. It was flying a Canadian flag. One of the biggest threats to our society was heading for Vancouver. A Death Ship! How many adults and children are sugar junkies in our country? Diabetes and obesity are at epidemic levels! How sad. There are natural sugars like stevia that are a far better choice.

**Chemicals.** Chemicals added to your food are unnatural toxic substances. They adversely affect your body and your brain in many ways. They disrupt the food's nutritional value. The food industry puts them in as preservatives. Products can sit on the shelf for years and still not spoil. But, these toxins sit in you. They don't necessarily leave. They stay in the fatty tissues of your body and your brain. This puts huge stress on you, suppresses your immune system and makes you more vulnerable to disease. It's a major reason why so many people get sick because their bodies are loaded with toxic chemicals. Does the food industry know this? Yes, of course. Your health and wellbeing are not the issues. Profit is. Making money is the motive. Business as usual. We are now in the 21$^{st}$ century and perhaps a central issue as to why this world is a suffering place for so many is the fact that THERE IS NO LOVE IN CORPORATE ECONOMICS.

Do you feel good? Are you mentally sharp? Our modern day eating habits are counterproductive. We eat too much of the wrong food. Does every order have to be large? What value is there in bottomless drinks and all you can eat venues? Say NO to large, you are paying to get fatter. Why eat a huge lunch and be sleepy the rest of the day? Empty caloric food was never part of our natural origin. Neither were tons of salt, sugar, saturated fats and thousands of chemical additives.

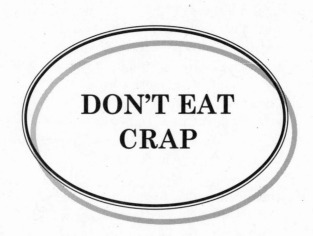

**DON'T EAT CRAP**

# 6.5 EXCITOTOXINS

**Excitotoxins**: substances added to foods and beverages causing brain cells to become over stimulated and die.

**Excitotoxicity**: a process that destroys neurons.

Excitotoxins are substances commonly used as food additives. They are found in all kinds of foods. These chemicals stimulate your taste buds. They make tasteless low fat foods tasteful. They are added to enhance flavour so that, you, the general public, will buy them.

Your brain is a chemical plant. It relies on quality control of chemicals to stay in operation. Since the brain receives blood continually from your body, it is exposed to chemicals all the time, some harmful, some beneficial. What regulates this is your **blood brain barrier**. This protective barrier controls chemical substances. Some are allowed to enter, others are excluded. Sadly, some excitotoxins are able to cross the barrier. When they do, neurons are stimulated to fire over and over until they are exhausted and literally "excited" to death.

For decades of my life, I listened to the tobacco industry **lie** and **deny** about how smoking cigarettes causes lung cancer and strokes. Finally, as you may know, there was enough indisputable scientific evidence piled up to the moon proving that smoking cigarettes does cause cancer. Today, there's no debate.

Here is an example of a warning contained inside a cigarette package from Health Canada:

> "*Can tobacco cause brain injury?*
> *Yes, it can result in brain injury.*
> *– Tobacco damages blood vessels and causes blood clots in the blood vessels of the brain.*
> *This causes strokes.*

*– Strokes often result in extreme disability, including*
*paralysis and loss of speech.*
*Strokes can also result in death.*
*– More than 2,500 people in Canada die each year from*
*tobacco-caused strokes.*
*Quitting smoking reduces your chance of having a*
*stroke."*

Huge class action lawsuits have occurred. Millions of people are sick from smoking tobacco and millions more have died from it. It's my opinion that the following food additives are in the same boat as tobacco. Big money is behind the denials of no proof, no proof. Profits come first. Sadly, millions of humans will have to suffer for a long time yet, until the truth is finally accepted.

There are three main excitotoxins used by the food industry. Most of us unconsciously eat some of them, everyday. Excitotoxins play a major role in degenerative brain diseases. Are you executing your own brain?

**Aspartame** is an artificial sweetener. It is totally man made and has no nutritional value. People can supposedly enjoy a product that tastes sweet but has no excess calories. But at what cost? More and more health experts, researchers, and doctors are saying that aspartame is dangerous for everyone. It slowly poisons people causing endless silent deaths. Aspartame is in over 1000 food products ranging from Diet products, to gum, to yogurt. The news is breaking through: Aspartame is clearly a chemical poison. I will never drink a can of Diet pop. It's too toxic. Aspartame has a very dark history. It's a scandal that it remains on the market. I encourage you to get more information about this insidious food additive.

**MSG (Monosodium Glutamate)** is a flavour enhancer. It is also a seasoning and filler in processed foods. There's no secret about this product. Many people are allergic to it. It makes them sick. I love to dine out occasionally. I frequent only restaurants that cook food with no added MSG. You should too. Before you serve the next can of soup to your family, see if it has MSG on the label. Before you cook your next pre-packaged dinner, check it out. If monosodium glutamate is written on the container, don't buy it.

**H.V.P (Hydrolyzed Vegetable Protein)** is used for flavouring and also as a food filler. It is added to soups, sauces and fast foods to give them a beef flavour. As well, H.V.P. is used to give a creamy texture to soups, sauces and dressings. This neurotoxin increases the production of free radicals in your body.

What an ironic situation! In general, the health profession is working to enhance our lives by developing methods, products and strategies to protect and heal us. Other groups in our society are making, promoting and selling excitotoxins as food additives that harm us.

The big question is whether or not these additives are necessary. So, isn't the best advice simply to stay away from them? Do not consume them. Do not feed them to your children or your grandchildren. They are not supposed to make you sick but they do. Many health conscious people are aware of these dangerous taste enhancers but the general public isn't. All citizens need to be educated about making safer, healthier choices. Be wise. Ask yourself: is this food additive healthy enough to become part of me?

## 6.6  WHY KILL THE 'CAPTAIN'?

The things we do on a daily basis naturally impact our health and wellbeing. Sadly, people are victims of their own ignorance. They are not aware about substances that can be toxic to the brain. A wise lifestyle avoids as many of the following substances as possible.

**Tobacco.** Smoking prematurely ages your brain. It causes blood vessels to constrict lessening essential blood flow to your most vital organ. Your memory is then compromised. Nutrients are deprived lowering the activity of the brain. Every cigarette smoked increases the number of free radicals in the body. Smokers are at a greater risk of dementia than non-smokers. Everyone should know the answer. **"BUTT OUT."**

**Caffeine.** Most of the caffeine consumed today is in coffee. There seems to be coffee shops on every corner. We are consuming more and more of it along with more sugar and more fat. Coffee has an upside and a downside. Yes, coffee will immediately stimulate your brain, wake you up, sharpen your mental performance, overcome fatigue and make you more alert. It can give you that extra boost, but you don't want coffee to be your primary source of brainpower. It is not a good idea to rely on it to get you going everyday. Coffee's downside is that it is a diuretic. It reduces blood flow to the brain. It puts you on edge in the fight or flight response. And when the effect wears off, you want more. The best practical advice would be to use it sparingly. Try drinking herbal teas instead.

**Prescription Drugs.** If you are taking any medications, check to see if there are any potential side effects. Medications can be brain toxic. They can affect the quality of your brain functioning. I highly recommend "The Better Brain Book" by David Perlmutter, MD. The hidden brain toxins in your medicine cabinet are exposed in his book. Consider finding non-pharmaceutical alternatives to prescription drugs.

**Alcohol.** Alcohol is a common brain poison depending entirely upon how much you drink. A glass of wine a week would be relatively harmless. Four or five glasses a day will increase your chances of dementia big time. Alcohol can cross the blood brain barrier contaminating the brain. Unfortunately, the blood brain barrier can't always keep poisonous chemicals out.

Alcohol depresses the brain, destroys the hippocampus and the all important dendrites. Scientists say that the prefrontal cortex is smaller and has fewer neurons in alcohol users. It's tragic to see so many people of all ages consuming alcohol. Brain scans of intoxicated people show that the 'Captain' isn't even on deck. No wonder it is against the law to drink and drive. Pregnant women, any age, should not drink any alcohol at all. The media glorifies it, the societal pressures are great, but the truth remains. Alcohol is toxic to your brain. Hangovers are considered funny to some people. The truth is that hangovers are brain damage. That's why they hurt.

**Street Drugs.** Street drugs are not harmless relaxing substances. There will always be debates and people will argue forever about their benefits. But, the fact is, drugs change your brain. Drugs change you. Marijuana is very harmful to the brain. Over time, abuse of it promotes chronic demotivation and puts holes in the brain. Cocaine, heroin, inhalants, LSD and ecstasy all destroy the brain and the person using them. Imagine a forest that has been burned by a forest fire. That's how scientists describe the brains of people who use Crystal Meth. It's a storm of <u>destruction</u>. If you watch an egg sizzling on a hot frying pan, that's what meth does to your brain.

What's the proof that tobacco, alcohol and drugs kill your brain? The new SPECT ( Single Photon Emission Computerized Tomography) brain scan equipment is absolutely fantastic. High-resolution, sophisticated brain-imaging techniques are on the leading edge of neuroscience today. These scans clearly show the damage caused by substance abuse. Proof is now available to us all. The brain destruction can't be missed. Abused brains look sick and toxic, like melted down candles. Brain scans are changing the world in which we live just like the first pictures of the earth from space did. Brain imaging represents a new horizon in human history and will emphatically alter the way we live forever.

Due to the effects of drugs and alcohol, the 'Captain', the prefrontal cortex of the brain, often isn't on deck. The widespread carnage inflicted upon the brains of so many unknowing people is appalling. The general use of alcohol and drugs is very harmful. The common label 'recreational drug' is an illusion.

A great resource is the Amen Clinic at www.brainplace.com. Check out "Images Of Human Behavior: A Brain SPECT Atlas". See for yourself. Holes in the brain are shocking to look at. Pictures don't lie!

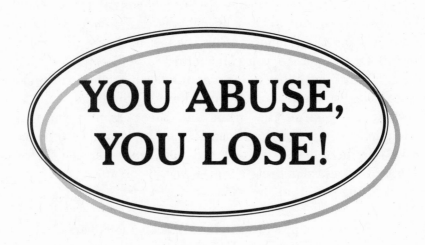

# YOU ABUSE, YOU LOSE!

# 6.7 TV ROTS YOUR BRAIN

We live in an electronic, worldwide village. Televisions seem to be everywhere. TV screens have just been installed in my local Credit Union. Small TV screens are now in some motor vehicles. Huge TV screens can be viewed while driving on the highways. Many homes have more than one television. People go on holidays or camp in the bush and take their screens with them. The media revolution has changed the way we live.

What television does to us is not fully understood. Television is not a simple machine. Images on the screen draw us like a magnet, hypnotizing us into a state that resembles sleep. There are many serious issues about viewing television.

Television can program you. It literally reinvents you. Too much television can make you "dumb". It bombards us with constantly changing streams of pictures, words, and fast, disconnected images. The brain gets exhausted from over stimulation. In order to survive the brain has to defend itself.

The brain's basic operation system is via pictures. People who make television programs know this. Have you noticed in the last few years how television images have speeded up? A great deal of programming contains more danger, threats or violence. A constant, never-ending stream of fragmented scenes bombards us. The result is chaos for your brain. You are put into fight or flight response. The 'Captain' is abandoned. Thinking stops. Your brain becomes overloaded because the images presented are too frightening for it. Television separates us from ourselves. It dulls the mind and the senses. Blank staring at the screen becomes the norm. Unfortunately, for too many people, the screen becomes the center of their world.

If you stare at the television screen for hours, your brain activity slows down. **You can become mentally passive.** The brain acts like a sponge soaking up all the images that it is exposed to. However, it is unable to discern or discriminate whether the images are having a positive or negative impact.

The muscles of your body grow weaker and smaller if you do not use them. The same happens when you watch endless hours of television. A lack of mental activity shrinks your dendrites; your prefrontal cortex gets thinner. You become the owner of a disadvantaged brain. Excessive television watching is basically a **NO BRAIN** activity. Our bodies and brains have not evolved by being inert creatures. The amount of time spent in front of a television screen is a monumentally significant issue.

Here's another way television steals your brain. The left brain is the logical, thinking, reasoning brain. It generates the language that we need to communicate. The current technology revolution is shifting us away from words to pictures and away from thoughts to feelings. Television stimulates the right brain that is specialized for emotions while shutting off the left brain. Thinking stops when you are emotionally stimulated. You are hooked and hypnotized. We are getting farther away from writing and reading. The shift is to the screen instead of books, magazines or newspapers.

Television sadly erodes our powers of attention and concentration. It weakens our natural powers. Observe and see how many people of all ages who cannot sit still, pay attention or focus on anything for more than a few seconds. These ADD (Attention Deficit Disorder) conditions are becoming more common and widespread. The need is to be conscious of how image based technology is detaching you from your left brain.

Finally, my experience for years teaching teens and adults has led me to conclude that television is a major cause of many learning and behaviour problems. Far too many people today live in an "<u>entertain me</u>" existence. So many people lack imagination and creativity. Interest in reading and writing are declining. Listening skills are poor. Television has provided bad role models and negative metaphors for life. Poor social skills are the result. Excessive television viewing produces and maintains BRAIN IMPROVISHMENT.

This is a HOT TOPIC indeed. Of course, some programming is excellent. There is no doubt about it. It's not all bad. Educational and knowledge networks make a wonderful contribution to our lives. Television can be a top-notch educational tool.

**Best Advice:** Ask yourself this question. "Will this program support me to become a better person?" Make intelligent choices. Choose programs that support you rather than belittle you. Choose building the brain over draining the brain. Avoid mind numbing, time wasting programs. It's your call.

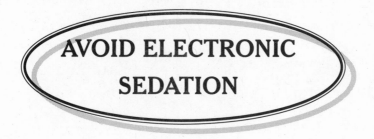

**AVOID ELECTRONIC SEDATION**

**Video Games**: Video games work on the pleasure centers of the brain. These games can be highly addictive. There are modest benefits. The drawbacks are greater. Unless, educationally oriented, they do not work the brain. So few games involve thinking, reasoning, planning or organizing. The 'Captain Of The Ship' can get depressed from endless, non-challenging repetition.

Video games dumb you down. No dialogue between people takes place. Players can become introverted and depersonalized. It's no surprise to hear researchers declaring that video and computer games slow down the progress of brain development for people of all ages. Learning occurs <u>only</u> in the very first minutes of playing a game. Then the brain growth stops and it is replaced by entertainment. A hundred hours of playing the game is like watching the same television show a hundred times. There is no benefit for the brain. What a huge waste of time.

**Violent video games are hazardous to your mental health**. Violence, rape, pillaging, gore all have a negative effect on you. They are harmful for your brain and your personality. They contribute to aggressive and anti-social behaviours. You can become a desensitized person by playing them. Isn't it crucial to stop any kind of game that changes normal functioning brains into malfunctioning ones?

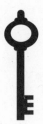 **KEY POINT:** Progressive educators and neurologists, among others, are treating TV and Video games as a public health threat. Have these sources of entertainment become the drug of the nation?

## 6.8 THREATS

The brain's number one job is to **survive**. Information coming into your brain that threatens your survival takes priority over all other information. When you are threatened, your old "reptile brain" immediately triggers the fight or flight syndrome. Stress hormones flood the body mobilizing it.

Did anyone ever threaten to punch your lights out? Here's what would happen. That potential hazard would send your defense system racing. Shooting into the center of your brain, the threat would stimulate the thalamus, your main relay switch. The fear signal would then be transferred to the amygdala activating your basic survival instincts. The brain would register: **danger! danger!** Conditioned reflexes happen quickly. Your thinking, reasoning frontal lobes would be shut down. This threat would put your brain on red alert. You would be ready to run away or fight to defend yourself.

Confrontations, difficulties, violence or excessive stress of any sort affect you negatively, hijacking your thinking brain. Your frontal lobes solve problems in your life. You need that 'Captain'. The conditioned reflexes of the reptile brain are necessary for survival as a last resort. If threats are dominant in your daily life, you will sink into a low level of thought and behaviour. It will be more difficult to pay attention, solve problems and perform higher order skills. You would be living in survival mode most of the time.

**KEY POINT:** Safe non-threatening environments are critical. Learning is inhibited by threats. You need to use your frontal lobes to eliminate negative threats and emotional stress.

# 6.9 VIOLENCE

If I am watching a movie and a violent scene is about to come on, I close my eyes. Violence upsets my whole system. It's not a pleasant experience for me. This common reaction can happen to you when you witness or take part in a violent act. Blood flow rushes to your brain and stress hormones flood in, enveloping your whole body. Violence makes your brain sick. Violence makes you sick as well.

Today, media violence is commonplace in a variety of programming. Even commercials on TV are becoming violent. The news mainly focuses on war and disaster. As we grow up, we are exposed to thousands of acts of violence via the media. **There are hundreds of studies indicating that media violence inspires real violence.** Aggression, mistrust, fear and suspicion are increasing. People are hooked on negative stimulation and becoming more desensitized. What is abnormal is becoming normal. The glorification of aggression, guns, and killing has to be eliminated if the human family is to survive.

Avoid violent movies or destructive games. Give a wide berth to profanity. Abstain from cruelty, fighting, killing, terrorism, and ugliness. Boycott these. Why pay money to degrade yourself? Violence activates your primitive brain and retards your growth as a human being. An anxiety-free brain is our birthright. Why waste it?

# 6.10 ALZHEIMER'S DISEASE

Alzheimer's (**AD**) is a progressive, degenerative disease. Several changes occur in the brains of people who have this disease. There is an accumulation of a protein called beta amyloid. Brain cells die or shrink and are replaced by this **plaque**. Plaque builds up in areas responsible for memory. A second sign is the existence of thread like **tangles** inside the cells. These tangles eventually strangle healthy cells. Brain scans show that the brain of a person with AD shrinks over time more than normal, affecting the efficiency of the brain. These conditions are not part of normal brain aging.

Generally AD develops with people over the age of 65. However, it can start much earlier. The term "early onset" means someone under 65 who is diagnosed with the disease. The biggest risk factor is age. Also, people who have a family member with the disease are at a greater risk than those having no history of it in their family. Scientists are investigating other factors. The environment is certainly high on the list as well as diet and a lack of exercise.

Most of us are aware that the effects of AD are literally devastating to the person who has it and everyone around them. It starts off with simple loss of memory. In the beginning we treat these experiences as absent mindedness or **senior moments**. But at some point conditions escalate. People forget where they live, the names of their friends and family members, where they put things, what they are supposed to be doing, more and more frequently.

The hippocampus (the memory center) is especially vulnerable to plaque. That's why memory problems appear first. Eventually, all aspects of your life are affected. Sufferers become isolated. They lose their will power. Hope fades. These degenerating changes in the brain will affect how you think, how you act and how you behave.

Presently there are over 400,000 Canadian seniors with dementia or AD. Estimates for the year 2030 remain at ¾ of a million. There are over 10 million baby boomers that are reaching the age when AD is most likely to manifest. There could be a potential tidal wave of affected people. That's very scary. Could you be one of them? I hope not.

Conventional wisdom says there is no cure. Yet, **THERE IS HOPE** to avoid this massive, imminent epidemic. Firstly, if you have noticeable memory problems, get medical help. Be proactive and support yourself, your family and your friends. Next, AD is not inevitable. The medical profession's approach is too passive. This brain disease cannot be reduced to one single cause that can be cured by one single pill. Society cannot wait for the 'miracle' cure. To prevent the AD wave, why not proceed under the hopeful banner that it can be delayed and even prevented. The answers and the hope for all of us lie in education. We need to learn to work and live in a brain compatible way. We need to focus on wellness instead of illness. The **plasticity** of the brain guarantees its youth and accompanying brainpower. Avoiding this cruel disease is the hope.

Help is available. Contact the Alzheimer's Society of Canada, www.alzheimer.ca. Prepare yourself. Don't let it happen to you. Don't just rely on the medical system or your Doctor. Rely on yourself. Be your own coach. This book offers dozens of prevention strategies. Be smart and implement them

> **Plasticity:**
> **constantly changing neurons have enormous potential to learn throughout an entire lifetime.**

now instead of claiming that problems aren't happening or it won't happen to me. Don't let arrogance be your downfall!

Brain cells can be referred to as trees. Healthy trees have lots of branches (dendrites). The trunk is strong and sturdy (myelin coated axon). There are lots of roots (synapses). As the years go by dendrites droop and fall off. The trunk withers and the synapses vanish. The trees disintegrate. In general, the brain reaches its peak around the age of 25. It begins its decline around the age of 30 to 35. Don't forget it is all relative to how you live your life.

(Diagram F)

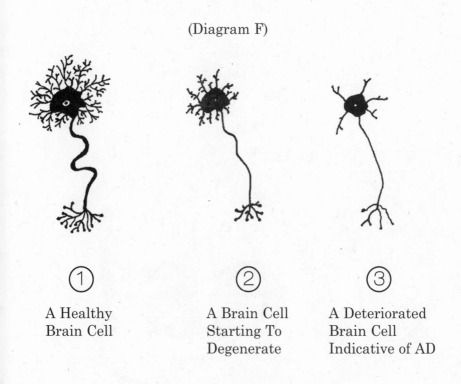

| ① | ② | ③ |
|---|---|---|
| A Healthy Brain Cell | A Brain Cell Starting To Degenerate | A Deteriorated Brain Cell Indicative of AD |

**Abundant brainpower means that your neurons are at Stage 1. No one wants to be at Stage 3. It's up to you. Grow those trees.**

Brain plasticity is the new frontier of hope. As you age, you have a choice between wellness and fitness or disease and pathology. Physical exercise is the most critical activity that affects the brain because it can slow down the degeneration of the nervous system. The ongoing effect of plasticity has to be also supported by the following:

- ☑ adequate hydration
- ☑ balanced nutrition
- ☑ adequate sleep
- ☑ good posture, flexibility and strength
- ☑ health problems under control
- ☑ healthy functioning heart, eyes, muscles and bones
- ☑ stress under control
- ☑ able to concentrate
- ☑ maintenance of a healthy weight

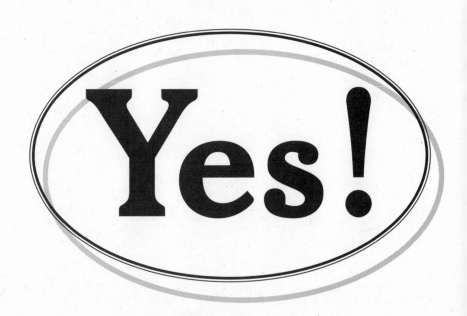

# Chapter 7

# Brain Boosters

Now for the GOOD NEWS! These twenty tips offer you practical advice on how to boost your brainpower through mental training. Obviously, you cannot do them all, but try something that attracts you. You choose. Don't forget, that your brain is totally UNIQUE. There are over six billion human brains on our planet and not one of them is exactly like yours. Go for what interests you. You are literally the architect of your own brain so start building a better brain today.

# 7.1 LEARNING

Learning is great brain medicine. A learning brain is a healthy brain. Learning keeps your brain active and alive. Learning increases your brainpower. Your brain is designed to learn new skills, new mindsets, new perspectives, etc.

*The brain is designed to process knowledge and information just as the digestive system is designed to process food or the lungs process oxygen. If food, oxygen or knowledge is cut off, the organism dies. It's that simple.*

*Richard Restak*
*Older and Wiser – How To Maintain Peak Mental Ability For As Long As You Live*

Why is learning good for your brain? The brain's operation depends upon the fundamental principle of **networking**. Absolutely everything you know is based on networking. No knowledge exists in isolation. Any one piece of information is **linked** to endless other pieces of information. Each and every neuron in your brain has the potential to form thousands of links to communicate with other neurons. This can give your brain the possibility of lighting up millions and millions of connections. Therefore, every time you learn something new, you are creating new linkages.

Your brain is like the World Wide Web. It has the potential to create an infinite number of connections. Whenever you learn something new, your brain has literally changed. The axons and synapses get bigger and stronger. There is more resistance to damage and aging. Also, neurons can communicate better with each other. They can get more efficient! They can store more information and retrieve it later. When you study, the pathways are enlarged and strengthened. If you can recall something that you recently learned, that obviously indicates that you have grown new links.

To develop a strong brain, you need to build as many pathways as possible. You need to use your brain to study, to learn, to gain new experience to build up your mental tools. Your intelligence involves constructing as many links as possible. Use those millions and millions of circuits in your brain. Build new ones to support the older ones. Don't allow your links to waste away, get weak and die. Keep your pathways young and efficient. Brain health depends upon **stimulation**. Your neurons function better if you have an active learning brain throughout your whole life. New learning is the key. Daily, repetitious activities do not benefit the brain as much as new ones do. New skills or knowledge create new connections that can help support the older ones.

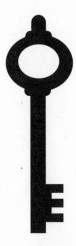

## KEY POINTS:

1. Some things are easy to learn while other things are very difficult. The key factor is **RELEVANCE**. If something is meaningful for you, it will be easier to master and it will stick in your long term memory bank for a longer time.

2. I'm sure you know you can learn anything whether it is hard or easy, if you have **FUN** learning it.

What happens if learning stops? If there is no new learning, the brain will gradually disconnect itself. Your overall mental capacity will decline. Your overall mental performance will decline. This can occur at any age. The brain gets weaker. The networks begin to fade and die out. If you do not feed the brain with learning, you will lose brainpower. A lack of mental exercise ensures shrinking brain cells and a gradual loss of brainpower.

**But am I too old to learn anything new?** No, you're not. You can enjoy and benefit from the brain's neuroplasticity at any age. As a Brain Coach, I assure you that it is never too late to learn something new.

Learning is the greatest brain booster we have at our disposal. It is never complete. You are on the right track if you dedicate yourself to learning something new all the time. Success in life depends upon it. Promise yourself, commit to yourself, and pledge to yourself that you will keep learning for the rest of your life. Start today.

**TO GROW YOUR BRAIN
YOU HAVE TO BE
LEARNING**

**IF YOU ARE NOT
LEARNING
YOUR BRAIN DOES
NOT GROW!**

## 7.2  LEARNING STYLES

Ways of receiving information are called learning styles. It is very useful to know your own personal learning style. There are three major learning styles.

**VISUAL**: These people tend to learn most efficiently by seeing. They learn best when they see pictures, movies, maps, diagrams, charts and by observing. They are often good readers and spellers.

**AUDITORY**: These people learn best by hearing. They prefer to learn through discussion, conversation, lectures, music, etc. They prefer to talk than write and would rather call you on the phone than write you a letter.

**KINESTHETIC**: These people learn best when they move, touch or do things. They don't like to sit for long periods of time because experiencing something first hand is essential for this type of learner.

You do not have just one learning style. We are more complex than that. For example, I am predominantly a visual learner. I need to see what is written, or what things look like. I need to draw something in order to understand it. I need a picture. As well, I am also a kinesthetic learner because I like to use my hands. I am not a strong auditory learner. Therefore, I consider myself to be a visual/kinesthetic learner. However, I do use all three modalities in my daily life. Most people do.

Since most of your brain is involved in every aspect of learning, we need to use all three styles as often as possible in our daily lives. That would make you a more responsible learner and boost your brainpower.

I highly recommend that you discover what your style is. On the Internet there are pages of learning style evaluations and questionnaires. Many of them are free. Do two or three to discover your style. Encourage your family and friends to do so as well. This knowledge can help you become more effective. Remember you can really improve your brainpower, and accelerate your learning if you:

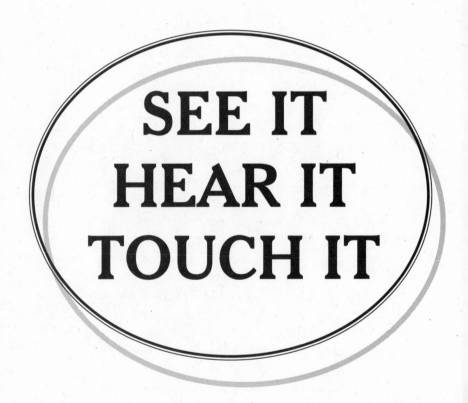

SEE IT
HEAR IT
TOUCH IT

## 7.3 LEARN ABOUT YOUR BRAIN

There is a new Renaissance in learning sweeping across the world today. It is being fueled by the exciting discoveries about the human brain. Throughout our long history, the brain has been a black box, an unknown, unrecognized mystery.

Guess what? If you are reading this book, you must be a brain owner. Therefore, because you own a brain, wouldn't you be interested in how it works? Your brain is fascinating to study. In fact, getting knowledge of how your brain works will literally make you smarter. The very best place to start boosting your brain is to learn about your brain.

Keep up to date. There are articles and stories about the brain popping up all the time. Stay sharp to catch the latest news about brain health. Changes are happening fast in the world and inside your brain. You want all the information and support you can get.

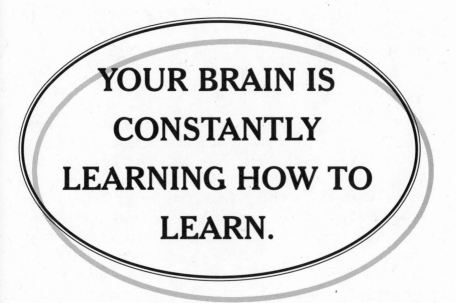

YOUR BRAIN IS CONSTANTLY LEARNING HOW TO LEARN.

# 7.4 EDUCATION NEVER STOPS

Your brain is literally a work in progress. It's never too late to learn. Every time you learn, you invest in your brain. If you learn lots of new things, you are establishing new circuits. If you don't, you are limited to using the same old connections. Are you mentally active or mentally inactive? When was the last time you had to learn something brand new?

Consider going back to school. Adult Education is available across the country. Complete your education. Further your education. Upgrade. Take a course in person or on line.

Community Recreation Programs offer a huge variety of things to try: swimming, sailing, CPR, gardening, cooking, mechanics, bookkeeping, dancing to name a few.

Elder College is open to anyone age 50-55 or older. The annual fee is minimal. Course tuitions are usually very affordable. Free seminars are often given. There are no tests or grades. Participatory learning is the theme. Courses, lectures and study groups are offered on a wide variety of topics. At the time of writing, Elder College in my community was offering courses on art, bridge, computers, literature, current affairs, social issues, history, science and agriculture.

Take a class on something that interests you. Better yet, take a course that is completely unrelated to your life. Put aside a few minutes a day to learn about something new. The more education you have, the less likely you will have problems as you age. Many studies clearly state that your level of education is a key predictor of longevity. Education increases the connection between brain cells. Education grows dendrites. Education maintains your mental abilities. The more variety of education you have over your lifetime, the less likely you will experience cognitive decline.

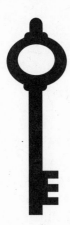

**KEY POINT:** The more education you have, the bigger your **brain reserve** will be. Your brain reserve means you have lots of information, knowledge and trillions of brain connections. It doesn't suggest that education will guard you against memory loss, for example, but it will give you the leading edge.

## YOUR BRAIN HAS A NEVER ENDING CAPACITY FOR LEARNING

# 7.5 COGNITION COUNTS

Who wouldn't like to be a little smarter? Wouldn't you like to be mentally sharp for the last days of your life? Cognition describes how your brain works.

Cognition is the process of knowing. Can you take action in your life? What type of thoughts do you have? How well can you concentrate? Are you able to solve problems? Are you alert most of the day or do you experience brain fatigue and fade out in the afternoon? Are you creative? Is your memory sharp? Can you rely on your memory? Do you have the brainpower you want? Do you have the brainpower you need?

Cognitive tools help you stave off brain decay. Protection comes from using your mind. Regardless of your age, take on mental challenges. Participate in a life of learning, thinking, problem solving and study. As you live your final decades, these pursuits will keep you mentally fit. The rewards of a mentally sharp life can't be understated.

Your personal cognition depends upon how well your brain works. So, can you increase your own intelligence, understanding, and awareness? **YES**. By your own attitude and effort, you and you alone can maximize your cognitive powers.

# 7.6 BRAIN STATES

All learning starts here. States are the condition of your body and mind at any given moment. There are learning brain states and non-learning brain states.

Here are some very common non-learning brain states: restlessness, boredom, apathy, confusion, frustration, distress, tiredness, anger or fear. The list is endless. There are literally hundreds. Some of these last a few seconds, others much longer. The key point is that it is difficult to learn in these states.

States are modeled in the outer world through our behaviours. Therefore, you can change your brain state if you change the behaviour. For example, if you are bored or tired you know that these are not the best brain states to be in. What can you do? The answer is totally obvious. **GET UP AND MOVE.** Movement, as you are aware, profoundly influences our brains, our bodies, our emotions and therefore our brain states.

Learning to manage your brain states is a key to longevity. You can affect your own brain state constantly. By being aware of your emotional conditions, you can switch from undesirable ones to desirable ones easily. Management can open you up to learning or if not, close you to learning. It can certainly make your life easier.

The cornerstone of effective living, learning and teaching is to always **ask questions**. Your brain is constantly trying to make meaning. Who, what, where, when, why, how? Get into question mode. Questions are to learning as an engine is to a car. Questions get your attention, bring answers and hence, meaning. **The brain wants meaning more than facts, info, theories or data**.

Ask a question and your brain will always look for an answer. Here's why. Inside your brain is a wonderful setup called the **Reticular Activating System**. When your brain receives a question, signals jump-start the RAS. This system pays attention. It pays attention because questions are relevant to it. Questions engage the RAS. Questions put us into THE NUMBER ONE BRAIN STATE for learning. This is hugely significant.

When it comes to learning, your brain is more receptive to questions than answers. Questions stimulate chemical reactions that promote learning and recall. When you ask yourself a question, your brain will continue to process it long after you have the answer. The search for the answer is far more powerful than the answer itself.

What is the best question to ask? The **"What if"** question. What if I became a genius tomorrow? What if I could grow a million dendrites a day? What if I could get a brain transplant? These "What if" questions put you into the future and put you into these superstar brain states:

- ◆ curiosity
- ◆ novelty
- ◆ challenge
- ◆ anticipation
- ◆ choices

Smart, brain compatible living means asking yourself at least one good question a day. By managing your own states on a daily basis, you will be open to a life of learning. Have you noticed how many questions have been asked of you in this book? Dozens. I hope every page is thought provoking enough to make you reflect on where your brain is at. Managing your brain states can make your life easier, not harder.

# 7.7  BRAIN WAVES

Your brain runs on electricity. Every single neuron discharges a minute electrical current. Millions of cells working together create patterns of electrical activity. These patterns are called BRAIN WAVES. Neuroscientists have divided them into four categories according to frequency. Think of them as radio frequencies, some higher or lower than others. Understanding these helps us to know about our own states of mind. This is very significant because it supports us to live and learn more effectively.

**Beta Waves**:

Beta waves are indicative of the state of mind during normal, awake, functioning, everyday activities. This is the state in which we spend most of our time everyday. Our eyes are open. We are walking around, working on things, talking, and generally focused on our affairs in our busy lives. We are concentrating, thinking, responding, and getting through the day. Beta is characterized by a high state of alertness.

It takes a lot of energy to be in a beta state all day. Our attention constantly shifts from one thing to another, as our brain has to deal with thousands of impressions all demanding its attention. If we function too long in a predominantly beta brain state, we can get tired, tense or stressed out.

**Alpha Waves**:

Alpha waves are slower than beta waves. If you close your eyes and start to relax, your brain waves will slow down. Alpha waves put you into a very relaxed state. There is no stress in an alpha state.

**Theta Waves:**

Theta waves are prominent when we are about to drift off to sleep. It is the state in which you are not fully awake and not yet fully asleep.

**Delta Waves:**

These are the slowest brain waves. You are technically asleep and most likely unconscious. Your heartbeat is very slow and your breathing is very deep.

Most people have no idea that it is possible to change brain states at will. Can you guess which state is the best for learning, for problem solving, for creativity, or for studying? ALPHA, OF COURSE.

You produce all four brain wave patterns all the time. The secret is that it is more beneficial for you to be producing more alpha waves than beta waves. A constant beta state can be very stressful and sometimes inefficient whereas an alpha state is far more relaxing and receptive. Your brain power potential can get a big boost if you can master a few simple techniques to put your brain on the right wavelength.

What's the secret? There is an intimate and significant relationship between our brain state and BREATHING. If you slow your breathing, you lower your brain activity. You can move from a busy beta state to a more relaxed alpha state by consciously changing your breathing pattern. **Slowing down your breathing is the most effortless way to alter your brain waves.** (See Breathing 4.3)

Other ways to produce alpha waves in your brain are: laughter, singing, chanting, daydreaming, listening to uplifting music, reading poetry, meditation, gardening, walking in nature, or enjoying something that you really like to do. Many

114

people call the alpha state "THE ZONE".

Taking a few moments everyday to slow down your brain waves is a top longevity secret. Alpha is a state of **"relaxed alertness"**, one of the foremost brain states.

**(Diagram G)**

## Your brain waves

**1. Beta**

**2. Alpha**

**3. Theta**

**4. Delta**

These are actual recordings of human brain waves
– from top:
1. When wide awake – the conscious mind,
operating at 13 to 25 cycles per second, the
so-called beta state.
2. The ideal learning state of "relaxed alertness," 8
to 12 CPS – alpha.
3. The early stages of sleep, 4 to 12 CPS – theta:
the mind is processing the day's
information.
4. Deep sleep, 0.5 to 3 CPS – delta.

The Learning Revolution, Gordon Dryden and Jeanette Vos, Ed.D., page 162.

## 7.8  CHALLENGE YOURSELF

For maximum brain growth, challenge yourself. Step out of your comfort zone and compete with yourself. Whatever moves you, go for it. Get out of the box once in a while and take a risk. Try something different. Anything that is stimulating to learn, exciting to try, new and different is certain to work your brain. Your brain gets challenged when forced to deviate from old established patterns. Your life as a human being is all about experience. If you are afraid of challenging yourself, take small steps. Do some simple things to start. After all, total lifelong comfort and security is not what life is all about. Exposure to challenge will keep you intellectually active and reduce your chances of developing dementia.

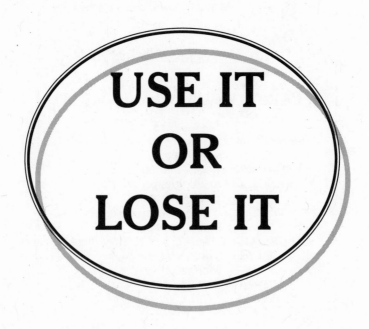

# 7.9 NOVELTY GROWS A BETTER BRAIN

How can you challenge yourself? The best way is through novelty. Novelty is good for improving learning and enhancing cognition. Unfamiliar activities are the brain's best friend. The brain is forced to pay attention. It gets more active.

The secret is to incorporate new and unknown experiences into your life because **your brain craves novelty.** Be creative! Be spontaneous! Travel to another country is a super star experience for your brain. You experience new and unfamiliar languages, money, food, customs, lifestyles, and climates, literally thousands of new things. Travel grows you as a person along with your brain. Two other wonderful top-notch novel activities are learning a foreign language and learning to play a musical instrument.

On a day-to-day basis, occasionally try rearranging your day, reconfigure your desk top, switch your furniture around, vary your work hours, take lunch at a different time, introduce some new art work to your office or new plants to your home. Every moment of our lives presents an opportunity to break our perpetual routines.

Did you know that monotony turns off your attention system? Unfortunately, dull, relentless, endlessly predictable routine doesn't give much stimulation. When important areas of your brain are shut down, it obviously interferes with your brain's ability to perform. Same old, same old, can be a killer. That's a fact and it is important to know that it does.

We do need predictable routines in our homes and on the job. Routines need to be maintained as part of everyday living. But, the secret is to occasionally slide a few novel experiences into those familiar routines. A little change is good now and then. CROSS TRAINING at work is an excellent strategy for any business. Learn several jobs and trade places with your fellow employees. Everyone benefits.

Why novelty? Your brain tends to focus on new and unfamiliar things. This is an ancient inherited trait from our ancestors who had to be perpetually alert to life threatening situations. The human brain is primed and on the look out to receive unexpected events. Novelty really turns your brain on and that's the way it has always been. Novelty stimulates dopamine which makes you feel good. Take advantage of that!

**KEY POINT:** Your brain has evolved to respond to novelty. Novelty keeps your brain fully functioning and alive, keeping the regulatory system for plasticity working. A lack of novelty can mean the brain can't perform its essential duties.

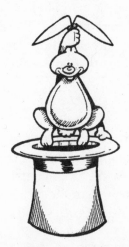

**Unless You Try To Do Something
Beyond What You Have Already Mastered,
You Will Never Grow!**

Cartoonist: Dave McCallum

# 7.10 READING GROWS DENDRITES

Reading energizes many areas of your brain. **YES**! The more you read, the more your neurons are stimulated to grow dendrites. Growing dendrites is a top strategy for brain wellness. You have to grow them continually to keep your brain in good shape.

The supreme benefit is that your memory gets better the more you read. Read an article from the newspaper, or a chapter in a novel. Then recall what the content was. Trying to remember strengthens the circuits in your hippocampus where memories are formed.

Read anything you can get your hands on: plays, drama, autobiographies, comedy, history, fiction, and non-fiction. Your local library has it all. No cost to you. Use that great resource. Remember we should all be grateful to have books to read, as many people in the world don't.

**What if I can't read?** Learn how. Find out what group or who can help you in your community. As well, ESL courses are offered coast to coast. Teachers are available.

**What if I don't like to read?** Now that you know that reading is one of the top brain boosters in existence, maybe you'll change your mind. Read small articles in magazines or newspapers and work your way up. The library most likely has audiotapes of popular and classic novels. Play the tapes and follow along with the book. As for some support, there are plenty of people who volunteer to help others read. It's all about attitude.

Taking a speed reading course will certainly grow dendrites. Work on building up your vocabulary. Another good strategy is to re-read a novel that you read years ago. Do you remember the plot? How about the setting? Have your impressions of the characters changed? How about your opinion of the novel? It's fascinating to see what your memory has stored away for all those years. Re-reading can really boost your self-esteem by simply showing you your inner strengths.

HERE'S A GOOD IDEA: Join a reading group. Better still, start one. There are hundreds of channels to watch but books are the best channel to tune into.

# IT'S CRITICAL TO KNOW
# HOW TO MAKE YOUR DENDRITES GROW

# READ, READ, READ, READ

# 7.11 WRITING JOURNALS

Journal writing is excellent for improving your brain. There are really no special qualifications for journaling. Just writing as you see fit is perfectly fine. Writing will help transform you into a more active learner.

Writing your thoughts down on a consistent basis is an excellent reflection tool. It helps to externalize your internal thoughts and feelings. By writing things down, it helps your brain organize and make sense of many pieces of information. As well, it increases your chances that the information will be retained in the brain's long term storage banks. Journaling definitely improves your memory.

Writing is a good way to solve problems. Because you have a written record, it can help you to relate to your present situation. It can help you improve your critical thinking. It can support you to come up with viable solutions. Writing your way through a problem supports cognition. Journaling is a brain boosting activity.

## 7.12 STORY TELLING

Story telling is more than a story. In fact, it is a special experience. In some ways, it is more powerful than reading. When you listen to a storyteller you are in a relationship with that person. You connect with the voice, facial features, hand gestures, body postures and a host of other living patterns. Listening to a detailed description gives your right brain a workout. Your auditory lobes are paying attention and your frontal lobes are working. You are very busy creating mental pictures in your mind. You are engaged in learning.

In my family, we read to each other frequently. My wife reads lots of long novels. She often tells the story to me chapter by chapter. I love that. My daily reality is suspended for a moment and I am transported into another world. Naturally, it stimulates discussion and more sharing.

My many years of teaching in the classroom have led me to this invaluable top secret. If you want someone's attention, tell him or her a personal story. It works like magic. We all love stories. Listening to stories or telling stories has always been one of the foremost ways to learn. Every culture in the world has a story telling tradition.

**KEY POINT:** Your brain is hard wired for story telling.

# 7.13 ART

Art is a powerful way to improve your brainpower. Here are three good reasons why. We live in a left brained world. We constantly judge, analyze, reason or problem solve. For balance, if we combine our left-brain world with more creative, intuitive right brain activities, we build links between both sides of the brain.

Another benefit is that art can fire up your brain and get things going. Art gives us a chance to be innovative and creative. It can lift us out of our comfort zone. Trying new pastimes helps us avoid mediocrity. Art can literally be personal enrichment.

As well, arts integrate your mind and body. The arts can link the way we think with moving and doing. It is a whole body activity. Painting, sculpting, pottery, ceramics, beadwork, sketching, costume design, dancing, acting, etc. are activities that literally build and sculpt a better brain.

Perhaps you are not so artistically inclined. Don't totally discount any of the arts. Learning about art is just as beneficial as participating in an art form. Go to a gallery. View an exhibit. Go to the library and take out books on art. Do it just for the experience. Having interest in some art form can be very stimulating and positive for your lifestyle.

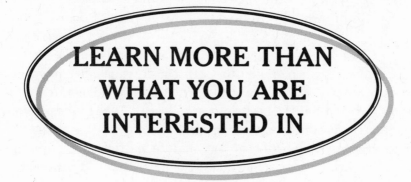

**LEARN MORE THAN WHAT YOU ARE INTERESTED IN**

# 7.14 MUSIC

Music has a powerful effect on your brain. Almost every-where you go today, music is playing in stores, malls, restaurants, office buildings, public events, sporting events etc.

We have all been hearing music since we were born. Music can move us in many different ways. It can help us heal or calm us down. It can inspire and lift us up. Music can lower our blood pressure and keep the blues away. Music activates our feet and our fingers, makes us rock our heads back and forth. Music literally makes us move. That's healthy because it propels us out of inertia by increasing our muscular energy.

Other ways music positively affects your brain are:

- Increases blood flow to your brain
- Counters fatigue
- Reduces pain sensations
- Relieves worry and stress
- Helps you feel good
- Stimulates thinking and creativity
- Improves concentration
- Improves memory
- Takes less time to learn

Everything you do involves your brain. If you knew that experiencing a certain type of music would be totally beneficial to your brain, wouldn't you want to listen to it? I do.

This music can get your brain doing a lot more for you. These sounds can help you to learn easier, remember more and produce at top performance levels. When the brain generates alpha brain waves, it has the best chances to learn. These sounds do that for you. The best learning systems in the world use this music. The beats are between 55-70 beats per minute, putting your brain into an alpha state of relaxed alertness. The music is called BAROQUE.

From the BAROQUE period (1600-1750 AD) has come the most highly recommended music. This music is generally simple. Mostly horns and strings are played. It has great value in promoting harmony and restful alertness. Here are some of the composers and their most famous compositions. These compositions are superb brain music, pure and simple.

Antonio Vivaldi – The Four Seasons
George Frederic Handel – Water Music
Johann Sebastian Bach – Brandenburg Concertos

The CLASSICAL music period (1750-1820 AD) was characterized by compositions that were full of energy and contrast. The first symphony orchestras were created. This music is also highly recommended.

Wolfgang Amadeus Mozart – Eine Kleine Nachtmusik
Ludwig Van Beethoven – Fifth or Ninth Symphony
Gioachino Rossini – William Tell Overture

You may have heard the idea that listening to Mozart "makes you smarter". The so-called Mozart Effect has been studied for over 10 years now. It is still controversial but there is a considerable body of evidence now declaring that Mozart's music (especially piano) improves cognitive functions.

**KEY POINT:** Even if you do not like Classical music, listen to it anyway. Buy yourself a Baroque CD. Play it once a day in your home or at the office so quietly that you can barely hear it. Your brain will glow like lights on a Christmas tree. Many, many areas of your brain will be engaged. It will put you into a positive relaxed state. It's awesome for your brain chemistry!

Here is an important issue about music choices. Listening to music activates the frontal lobes of your brain. It has a positive influence on your heart rate, immune function and stress levels if you find it to be pleasant. So, if you do not like a certain type of music, you should not listen to it. It will turn off key parts of your brain. Heavy metal and acid rock music are not recommended as beneficial music for good reasons. It can be emotionally disturbing, shut down thinking and decrease serotonin production. Of course, music choices are highly personal. We are all encouraged to make wholesome music choices.

Any kind of musical training stimulates our brain circuits as well as creating new ones. It is highly beneficial to learn to play a musical instrument especially if you are a middle-aged person or a senior. With proper instruction, almost anyone can learn to play music.

Everyone has a favourite song. Songs make us happy. What's your favourite song? When you sing or hum or listen to a song you like, your serotonin and dopamine levels are elevated. You are emotionally engaged, feeling good, maybe even inspired. Your brain is awake and your body is energized. Enjoy!

(Diagram H)

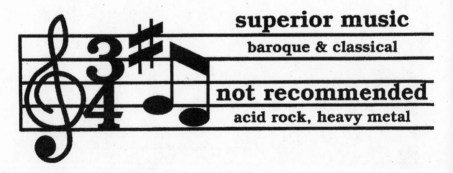

superior music
baroque & classical

not recommended
acid rock, heavy metal

Your Magical Brain How It Learns Best, Gary Anaka, Portal Press, 2005.

# 7.15 PROBLEM SOLVING

Tune up your brain with puzzles. There are lots of different ones: crossword puzzles, word searches, sudoku puzzles, crostic puzzles, riddles, brainteaser questions and many more. They can be found in the newspapers or, if you go traveling and you are near a bus depot, train station or airport, pick up one of those inexpensive variety puzzle books. These books are worth their weight in gold.

Doing puzzles have benefits that show up on aptitude tests. Crossword players do very well on verbal tests. Jigsaw enthusiasts score well on spatial reasoning tests. Bridge players perform best on memory and strategy tests. Forget bingo. Do a puzzle.

Puzzles and mind training exercises are flooding the market. As bodies age, the mind can go with it. Games and puzzles are popular because they are promising brain builders according to researchers.

Puzzles and games will help you but they are not medicine. It's hard to say that a person who does 5 sudoku puzzles a week is ahead of someone who only does 1 a week. It is just not known how much puzzles can help you avoid dementia later in life. But they do provide challenge and stimulation that the brain craves. Puzzles are also superb teaching tools for people of all ages.

Some time honoured top-notch games are chess, checkers, jigsaw puzzles, bridge, scrabble or Rubik cubes. Try to play occasionally with people who are better than you. They can push you to improve.

My top pick of all would be MENSA books, puzzles and games. I have used them personally and professionally for years and I highly recommend them to anyone. There are always lots of Mensa puzzle books around my home. I really enjoy my daily Mensa puzzle tear off calendar. Mensa is a worldwide society that exists entirely for people who like to think, learn and use their brain. Check them out.

*A list of Brain Training Companies and their programs can be found in the Resources section at the back of the book.

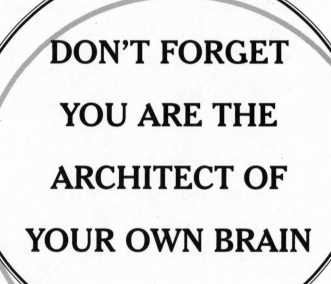

DON'T FORGET

YOU ARE THE

ARCHITECT OF

YOUR OWN BRAIN

# 7.16 MATH CALCULATIONS

Our reliance on machines is not always in our best interest. How often do we reach for a calculator when we need to multiply two numbers together or add a few numbers? Doing calculations in your head or on paper is good for you. Many parts on both sides of the brain are activated when solving simple math calculations. Most importantly, when you do a math problem the prefrontal cortex is thinking and learning. Solving on paper with a pen or pencil is far superior to pressing a button on a calculator.

*Learning is experience.*
*Everything else is just information.*

*Albert Enstein*

# 7.17 USE YOUR HANDS

Your two hands are the antennae for your brain. Using your fingers and hands keeps your brain alive. You don't always have to use a machine. Nothing wrong with doing things by hand! If you have a dishwasher, give it a rest and try washing the dishes by hand once in awhile. Give your leaf blower a break, use a rake. One of my longevity goals is to eventually downsize my lawn mower to a simple push mower. Many of our longest living Canadian women sew, needlepoint, crochet or knit. Craftwork is super. Making models, constructing things, repairing things are excellent brain boosters for men or women. Keep your hands busy. Any activity involving manual skills supports the brain.

Pick up a pen and sign your name with your non dominant hand. This will activate the other side of your brain. It's good to do things that feel unnatural with your hands. If you are right handed, try eating a meal, brushing your teeth, buttoning your shirt or clicking with the mouse with your left hand. Using your non dominant hand makes the opposite side of your brain access unused brain circuits. These would be new behaviours that the brain doesn't normally participate in. These types of simple exercises create new connections and expand your circuits.

There is a new science of brain exercises called NEUROBICS (Keep Your Brain Alive by Lawrence C. Katz, Ph.D. & Manning Rubin). Neurobics involves using your five senses – touch, smell, hearing, taste and sight. Our senses need ongoing stimulation to support a strong memory. Neurobics recommends different lifestyle choices to strengthen your brain connectors and gain new sensory experiences. Fun and novelty are the keys. Here are a few of the types of things to do besides using your other hand to give your brain a beneficial workout: do a routine task with your eyes closed, take different routes to work, look for unusual signs or landmarks, bring new smells into your life with soaps, teas, or essential oils, sample exotic fruits, enjoy a silent meal, occasionally wear ear plugs or eat different spicy foods. Neurobics strongly advocates using your creativity to break out of your daily routines. New multi-sensory experiences get your brain going and growing. The opportunities to stimulate the sensory areas of your brain are endless.

**A good story** – After 20 years of presenting workshops, here's one of my favourites. I did a keynote presentation at an all women's Conference some years ago. I was sharing about the NUN study in the United States. Over 3,000 Roman Catholic school sisters, all born before 1920, donated their brains after they died to a long-term study of mental decline and healthy aging. The nuns were known for their remarkable memories. I described their lifelong habits and simplistic way of living which involved lots of hand labour. The point I want to illustrate was that these nuns might represent the last of a traditional, technologically free way of living. When I asked for questions, a lady hollered from the back of the room "I know why these women had such good brains. They never lived with men!"

## 7.18  INCREASE YOUR BEST SKILLS

What are you good at doing? What do you like to do? Many activities we do at work or at home involve repetition. You simply have to do them over and over, day in, day out. There is no escaping it. That's the way life is. However, look toward improvement. Try to get better at what you do. Expand your abilities. Learn more about being more proficient, or quicker or improve your techniques. Try a little harder. Push your limits – that can help keep your brain healthy.

# YOU HAVE A TOTALLY UNIQUE BRAIN THAT HAS BEEN CUSTOMIZING ITSELF SINCE THE DAY YOU WERE BORN

# 7.19  MIND MAPS

Mind maps are truly one of the best learning tools ever invented. They are simple, easy to do mental models that make learning easier. Anyone of any age can make one on the spot, anytime, anywhere in no time at all. They are the best way to use your memory. They are super for planning, problem solving, studying, predicting, reviewing and making speeches. They help your brain understand the situation while literally encouraging higher order thinking. Mind maps support you to use your brain to its fullest potential. A great bonus to making a mind map is that they are fun to do.

A mind map is a drawing. Mind maps put your thoughts on paper giving you an overall picture. They graphically represent whatever ideas you are learning or working with. Why do they work so well? A mind map reflects the organizational predisposition of the brain. It reflects the actual biological structure of your brain because your brain thinks in pictures! They are like models of your neurons. Drawing a mind map taps the brain's greatest capacities.

## HOW TO MAKE A MIND MAP:

Draw a circle or any shape the size of an egg in the middle of a piece of paper. Print the idea or concept in the circle. This gives you a central focus. Then, draw your way out. Make branches radiating out from the main concept with ideas that relate to your concept. Then, make sub branches with smaller details or key words. Do your own thing. Let your imagination guide you. The key is to create visual emphasis. Use lots of colours, pictures, arrows, branches, indicators, symbols, or doodles to help stick ideas into your brain. This is a free form method of outlining.

I used mind maps with students for many years. They work! They can get you started. They can get you unstuck. They are a generic power tool that is one of the best brain boosters of all. I use simple ones in my life all the time. Think with a mind map.

(Diagram I)

## A Two Minute Mind Map

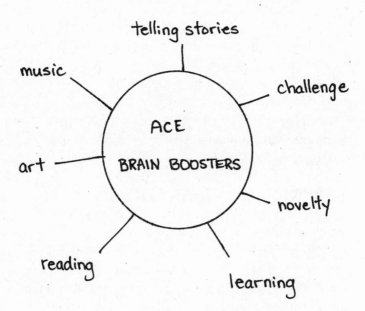

# 7.20 STUDY TIPS

(Diagram J)

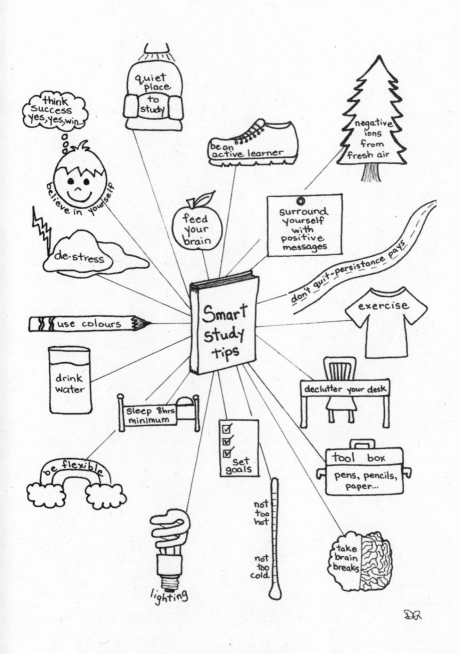

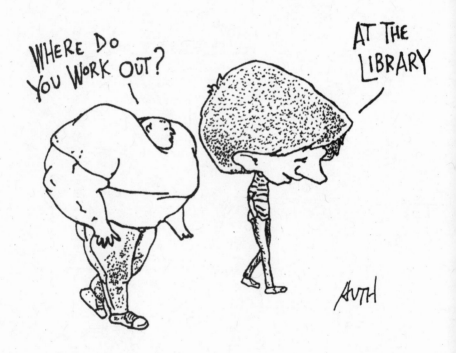

Cartoonist: Tony Auth

# CHAPTER 8

# Brain Compatible Lifetstyles

Life without a functioning brain is meaningless. Yet, most of us spend more time combing our hair than thinking about our brains. The following lifestyle suggestions offer practical support and will help you maintain your brain wellness program. There are no miracles, but your lifestyle decisions made on a daily basis add up over time in a big way. These are major players in your life. They make the difference between a brain remaining sharp as you age or a brain that goes fuzzy. Put them into action. Here's how to live in a brain compatible way and shape your brain's destiny.

# 8.1 MID-LIFE BRAIN POWER

Life is a paradox. It is true that as you get older there may be losses. Learning new things could gradually get harder, remembering can become a bigger challenge, and your brain-power could get feebler. "Losing your marbles" or "you are not all there" are the old stereotypes. Not very nice, but those could be the realities. Stop! You have a choice. Accept those old stereotypes and just sit for the rest of your life, or remain alive and vibrant.

You do not have to endure those negative fates. Life does not have to be all downhill with aging. The times have changed for the better. There are **big dividends** for you as you approach your midlife years because that is when your mental powers reach their peak.

Perhaps one of the greatest gains of aging is **WISDOM**. Wisdom is certainly one of the best and most desirable traits a human being can have. Living many years has the potential of providing you with this positive asset. With every year you have lived, millions and millions of dendrites have sprouted making trillions and trillions of connections. Their extensive networks only got there after a lot of accumulated knowledge and experience. Wisdom is the prize you get for living a long time.

Younger people in human history have tended to be our radicals, rebels, movers and shakers. Older people have been our greatest minds, inventors, teachers, philosophers, and writers. Martin Luther King, Nelson Mandela, Mother Theresa, and Gandhi were all very intelligent but it was their wisdom that made them great.

The reasons for being wise are many as you reach mid-life. With a healthy older brain, you can exercise better judgment. A lifetime of experience has given you better problem solving skills. You can offer fair council, mentor others, provide a deeper understanding and insight to life's challenges. You can be the prophet who tells stories to pass on knowledge, beliefs and customs of your culture! You have more time to listen. You can play a host of different roles that younger people aren't able to provide. You have survived your years of living so that you can support others with great intelligence.

I want to repeat the exciting news. The slow loss of brainpower as you age in your daily life doesn't have to happen. Researchers are revealing many hopeful discoveries. As we age, new systems come on line. Older brains can actually rewire and reorganize themselves. Don't forget, it is a fact that you can grow new brain cells throughout your whole lifetime. Mature brains will continue to produce new brain cells as well as endless new connections. Don't buy the old standard notion: older means worse.

Another great occurrence is that the two brain hemispheres begin to work better as a team. That's a fantastic upgrade in the management system. What can older brains do that younger brains have trouble with? They can see the bigger picture. An older adult watching a soccer game would generally be good at picturing the flow of the entire game, whereas, a younger person would be focused on an individual player. Aging makes a big difference on how the brain operates providing you with a lot of positive benefits.

Finally and most helpful of all, is the certainty that you **can** teach an old brain new tricks. <u>YES</u>! **The aging brain has great resiliency.**

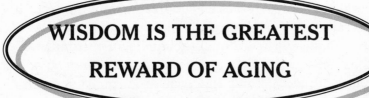

# WISDOM IS THE GREATEST
# REWARD OF AGING

# 8.2 MULTITASKING MANIA

In today's world, it is probably safe to say that almost everyone has to do some multitasking. I am sure you have noticed that younger brains seem to be able to do a lot of things at the same time. Younger people can multitask easier and absorb information very quickly because younger people are wired differently. They have been raised with technology their parents never had and have trained themselves to use it.

Older brains have more problems with multitasking as the brain begins to gradually change with age. Multitasking definitely can become a problem.

Women are naturally better at it than men. They are able to do many things at once. Men are at their best when they do one thing at a time. People have always been multitasking but not like today. Today's world is full of intrusive technology. In the past, it was easier to keep centered and in control.

**Your brain is designed to do one thing at a time**. It is impossible to do two things at once. What we are doing is switching our focus back and forth from one thing to another. We think we are doing more than one thing at a time but we are not. This is because we are moving so fast between the two. It does not matter if you believe this or not. **Repeat: You can only do one thing at a time**.

Here is today's great challenge. You can be in your kitchen stirring soup, feeding the baby, listening to the radio and sweeping the floor all at the same time. This can easily be done because these activities do not involve thinking. Your little brain (cerebellum) is in control and does them for you. However, if you're trying to write an email, complete an overdue year-end report, balance your budget and decide on some new equipment to purchase all at the same time, you are using your prefrontal cortex. That's a considerable challenge! Those are front of the brain thinking activities. This is how the 'Captain of the Ship' gets overloaded, tired or stressed out.

## WE ARE NOT MACHINES WE CANNOT ENDLESSLY PROCESS TASKS

I retired early from teaching because I realized that my brain could no longer endure the intense multitasking that was required to do my Special Education job. I had been a proud addicted multitasker for nearly 30 years. I loved to "get things done" and to support hundreds of students every year. I craved the buzz of adrenaline and dopamine in my brain. Why just teach two special programs at once when I could teach three? Inevitably, the drawbacks began to pile up. I could never keep up. Too many kids with too many problems. I began to feel that it was my fault I was behind. I also began to feel inefficient and gradually I lost one of my top qualities – patience. Nervousness and panic arrived with me on the job. I worked on channel overwhelm. Finally, the greatest enemy of the modern workplace took its toll on me. **INTERRUPTIONS!**

You should know what I am talking about. Interruptions at home or at the workplace consume vast amounts of our time and energy. Those enticing gadgets can really shackle us. Other people can too. Our thoughts get disrupted. Our concentration is broken. Interruptions make us less efficient. Tasks take longer because of diversions. Often, tasks aren't done as well because our efforts are fractured. Constant mental switching that goes on impairs our ability to think clearly. It also affects how we function overall as human beings.

Here's some practical advice to get a little control back into your life. Firstly, why not just TURN IT OFF. Why not just shut it down for a while? Wherever I go in my hometown or wherever I travel, I see endless numbers of people displaying their cell phone addictions. Talk, talk, and talk! Check, check, check! That's dopamine at work. Addiction to Internet activity is the same. Do you have to take that blinking BlackBerry to bed with you? Yes, we are super busy but we have to stop fooling ourselves. Are we being driven to distraction? Constantly shifting attention has consequences. There is a plague of attention deficit disorder especially in the work place. Unplugging is becoming a requirement for survival. Don't let multitasking become your personal extreme sport.

Secondly, the case for doing one task or project at a time is very strong. That's the way your brain naturally works. That's smart. **Unitasking** instead of multitasking is a good survival strategy.

Finally, a bit of time needs to be invested in periodic breaks. There is a real need to be free for a few moments just to think, relax, or internalize to avoid overload.

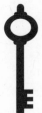 **KEY POINT:** As we age, multitasking becomes more challenging. So, it is very important to shut down distractions, focus and really concentrate on what you are doing.

# 8.3 SPEED KILLS

This is fast track, fast lane 21$^{st}$ Century living. We drive like crazy. Yellow traffic lights have become green lights. We cut our holidays short or we don't even take holidays. Working on weekends is normal. It's now a 50-hour work week. We stay up late. We don't read books or newspapers because it takes too long. We say hello to our 4 year old in the morning with a sticky note on the fridge door. We eat breakfast in our vehicles. We brush our teeth and text a message while we sit on the toilet. We have too many things to do. We are overscheduled/overbooked. The tasks are endless. Going slow tends to bug us. We can't wait to do the next thing. It's go, go, go! We are ready to snap.

Are you a speed addict? Have you become enslaved by technology, machines, laptops, cell phones, the Internet? The love of speed seems to have captured us all. Work has taken over our lives. We have become human doings instead of human beings.

"Stop the bus, I want to get off" is a common feeling for many professionals and people in all walks of life. I hear so many complaints about the frenzied pace of life. Too busy. Not enough time. I have to get through the day, week, month. Here is an honest question to ponder. "Do you feel that you are just getting through life rather than living it?" Making a living and having a life are not the same thing.

I am a recovering **workaholic**. As a Special Education teacher, that was the name of the game. Endless kids to help, lessons to prepare, meetings with parents, staff meetings, track practice, environment club activities, preparing report cards, behaviours issues etc. This went on year after year and I loved it. I enjoyed the delights of speed. My brain chemicals were wired for action. I was hooked.

I suffered from "time sickness". There just wasn't enough of it even in the summer. I was part of our attention deficit society. My social economic position in life was pushing me to go faster. As the pace increased and the years went by, I realized that this was a huge problem. Working like mad gave me my identity and a lot of intense good feelings. But, I was beginning to slowly **BURN OUT**.

With my training and work in Applied Neuroscience, I could see the writing on the wall. One of the hardest things to do in life is to change your mind. I had to. I was low on energy and getting health problems. I began to recognize my loss of brainpower. It became harder to focus! Life was overwhelming. I had to decelerate. I was manifesting the exact symptoms of brain degeneration that I teach people about in my workshops.

Burnout is a great teacher. I have personal friends, colleagues and acquaintances that have burned out. It's no joke. They lived mega hyper speedy lives. They avoided themselves and just kept going. They were in denial. Are you?

Look around you. How many of us are stressed out, soon to be burned out? Hundreds of thousands of Canadians have brain problems or brain diseases right now. What has gone wrong? Why are we constantly stuck in fast forward? Something must be missing. What's the mysterious answer? It is as obvious as the nose on your face.

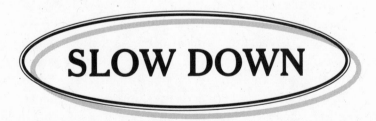

**SLOW DOWN**

Yes, technology has brought us fantastic labour saving devices. It has changed our work world and our lives. Life is better or is it? We have ended up being busier. And that's a FACT.

For many of us, our lives have become DISCONNECTED. We have lost touch with our children, family, friends and ourselves. We have lost connection to our food, to the places we live, to our planet and to life.

Our fast paced life has brought us to accelerated brain aging. We push our bodies beyond healthy limits and we ignore our inner voice that whispers "SLOW DOWN".

Rejoice! Societal values are starting to shift and changes are happening. More and more conscious people don't want to live speedy lives anymore. They crave sanity and harmony. They want to be more connected to living. Changes are slowly beginning to manifest. The Slow Food Movement is a prime example.

The simplest solution for our speedy way of living is to pay more attention to how we live. The secret is to try to live **mindfully**. Be aware of your present behaviours, habits and attitudes. Be open to experience life in the present moment, whether good or bad, pleasant or unpleasant. That's where the magic of life lies because the only time we really have is the present moment.

# 8.4  VOLUNTARY SIMPLICITY

There are many views and definitions about what voluntary simplicity is. I am not referring to politics, religion or technology, nor a life of poverty.

We all live in a fast, electronically complicated world. Life is a 24/7 experience. We are overloaded with work, anxiety and stress. These conditions seem to be contagious. So many people are sick and unhappy.

The bottom line is whether or not we are too preoccupied with money and material things. Too much never seems to be enough. We own too many things – our stuff controls us. The relentless quest for more, bigger and faster is not only killing the planet, it is killing us. Underlying this is the question of **brain sustainability**. Can your brain last with the continuous stressful pressure or will it collapse?

You choose the lifestyle you want to live. Voluntary simplicity implies that you live an examined life. What is important to you, what do you value or support? Your choice of appropriate lifestyle is about living in a brain compatible way. You can either enhance or reduce your brainpower by the way you live.

> *To be satisfied with a little, is the greatest wisdom; and he that increaseth his riches, increaseth his cares; but a contented mind is a hidden treasure, and trouble findeth it not.*
> *Akhenaton*

Living more simply is a source of wisdom we need to regain.

# 8.5 AT WORK

Do you ever experience brain fog at work? Do you ever have a project to do and your brain is just too dull to do it? You just can't seem to get into it. That has a lot to do with how your brain works. You can be "**stuck**" in the wrong place.

Your brain operates on the <u>Right/Left Dominant Cycle</u>. This cycle operates on 90-minute periods 24 hours a day whether you are awake or asleep. At any given time, your brain is very active in one hemisphere while the other hemisphere is taking a rest. Every 90 minutes they switch.

Here's the problem. Suppose you need to write a report. That means you need to access the left brain where language is stored. However, at that moment, your brain activity just happens to be in the right brain. That means you don't have access to language. Your active right brain is busy doing something completely different. No words or vocabulary are available. That's a problem making it very difficult to make any progress on that report.

Conversely, if you need to come up with a new idea or create something new but your left brain happens to be dominant at that moment, it will again be hard to get results. The left brain is not responsible for creativity, pictures or images. The right brain is. Your brain is stuck again. What to do?

The solution is obvious – **get moving**. Ideally you want to have both sides of your brain working. Stand up and do some cross lateral exercises, walk around, stretch or stand on your toes several times to get your whole brain activated. Movement for just a few moments will get your brain unstuck keeping your productivity levels up while on the job.

# 8.6  BEST TIMES OF THE DAY

I am a morning person. I love to get up early all year round, usually between 5:30 – 6:00 am. Here is the best use of my personal brain clock for a typical day. It parallels the best general patterns suggested by researchers. See if they match your daily routine.

| | |
|---|---|
| 6:00 – 9:00 am | very good time for creativity, ideas, inspirations |
| 9:00 – 12 noon | best time to solve problems, think, brainstorm, make decisions, excellent productive time |
| 12:00 – 3:00 pm | low brainpower, poor concentration, afternoon downtime needed, do routine chores, physical work, exercise |
| 3:00 – 6:00 pm | second round of production time |
| 6:00 – 8:00 pm | regenerating the brain, exercising, reading, do physical activities |
| 8:00 – 9:30 pm | not a good time for mental work, hard to concentrate, need to slow down the brain, stop stimulation and sensory input |
| after 10:00 pm | sleep – brain does its housekeeping chores |

There are two times of the day available for peak mental performance for me. I schedule my workday around these realities doing other activities when my brain batteries are lowest.

Naturally, everyone is different. If you want to maximize your brainpower potentials, discover your own brain clock. Become aware of your patterns and what times work best for you.

If you are a nighthawk, you would naturally wake up later. The first few hours of the day aren't usually your best time, which means your best creative times would be different from mine.

Be smart and pay attention to your personal brain schedule. Have meetings at times when you are most alert. Make significant decisions during peak mental times. Don't waste your best hours doing mundane, routine tasks that do not require a lot of brainpower. Be smart and use your natural brain clock wisely to take advantage of your best times of the day.

**Brain Fitness Exercise** – I have owned a watch for many years but I rarely wear it. At home or when I travel, I love to play this game. Guess what time it is? Since I was a teenager, I have enjoyed guessing the time. It's a way of keeping my brain engaged and focused in the moment. I feel really good when I am able to guess within a few minutes of the actual time. I do this virtually everyday. It helps keep my brain sharp.

## 8.7 YOUR SOCIAL BRAIN

There is a mountain of research proving over and over again, that a strong network of family and friends is essential for our well-being. It makes survival sense. We live longer, function better, heal from illness faster and keep our cognitive faculties longer. No man should be an island unto himself.

Social Neuroscience is a new field of study. It is a big deal in terms of understanding how our social experiences change the brain. It's all about our relationships and interactions with other people in our lives. It influences all of us. Our brains change in response to our engagement with others. A healthy amount of contact with our family, neighbours and colleagues means a healthy brain. Nurture your social brain.

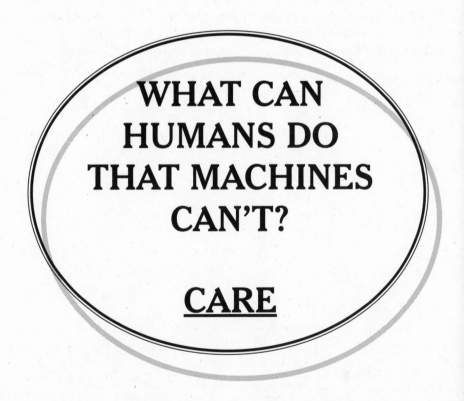

**WHAT CAN HUMANS DO THAT MACHINES CAN'T?**

**CARE**

## 8.8 DECISIVE ROLE MODELS

Who is your hero? Heroine? Positive role models are essential in our lives. Sadly our popular culture glorifies stupidity all too often and, unfortunately, anti-intellectual fools are on display on television and in the movies. They promote the impression that it is cool to be dumb. Avoid that like the plague.

A new area of research in neural science centers around the discovery of "mirror neurons". When you watch someone doing something, a network of neurons fires in your brain in the same way as if you were actually doing it yourself. In other words, we copy other people's movements and behaviours and learn from them.

Keep your personal mentors in focus. Look for inspiration. Look for leadership and integrity. Allow people like Terry Fox, Rick Hansen or Craig Kielburger to motivate you. The best teachers in life are good role models. Pick uplifting and supporting ones.

**KEY POINT:** Role models provide us with metaphors for life.

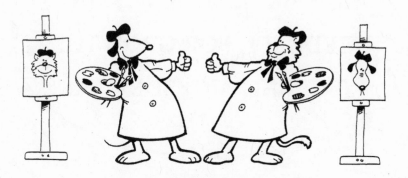

**People Need More Models Than Critics!**

Cartoonist: Doug McCallum

## 8.9 FEEDBACK

The brain thrives on feedback for growth, learning and survival. Your brain needs it and so do you. We all do. Feedback keeps us motivated. On going, continuously positive feedback is a must for our health. We need feedback daily to feel that we are doing okay. Feedback is a wonderful tool providing incentive if we are trying to break a bad habit. It can also help establish action plans. Surprises, rewards and praise can provide excellent feedback.

We need feedback at work if we are learning new skills. We need feedback in our relationships with our family and friends. Feedback can be as direct as the response to the question "How am I doing?" or it could be a group discussion, peer edit, employer review, a checklist or chart that displays our progress. Feedback gives us those little victories we need to stay positive. Learning is supported and your brain reaps the benefits.

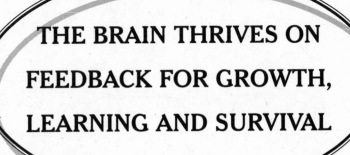

THE BRAIN THRIVES ON FEEDBACK FOR GROWTH, LEARNING AND SURVIVAL

# 8.10 BENEFICIAL RITUALS

Rituals are good to have in your life because they make us feel safe. The brain does not learn and grow if it is threatened. Rituals can be simple or elaborate. They can be daily, monthly, seasonally or yearly. Rituals are a form of established ceremony or behaviours that are repeated. Shaking hands is a common ritual. Hugging is another. In my workshops I have several rituals. I always play uplifting music before starting, everyone is invited to do brain gym to wake up, and "yes claps" always end my sessions. People like and appreciate these opening and closing rituals.

Having some regular rituals in your personal life and in your workplace is a very intelligent activity to pursue. Rituals are the regular rhythms of life. The sun rises and sets, the seasons come and go, the days and years pass by orchestrated by the great rhythm of life whether we realize it or not. Plants and animals are governed by instinctive rituals. Even your body has its own natural rhythms. Obviously your brain has a natural tendency for them. Because we live in a world that is rapidly changing and often in conflict, rituals help us to feel calm, wholesome and connected.

# 8.11 AVOID BRAIN INSULTS

**Concussion**: a stunning, damaging or shattering effect from a hard blow or collision; a jarring injury of the brain resulting in a disturbance of cerebral functioning.

Your brain is a delicate little bag of mush with the consistency of medium-firm tofu. It is soft and very vulnerable. Unfortunately, it can easily be injured. Concussions are a common occurrence in sports, on the job or at play.

When you hit your head with force, the brain gets bruised. And, it gets bruised again when it collides with the lining of the skull. Your neurons get scrambled and your neural networks get torn, broken, stretched and disconnected. A better description for a concussion is brain damage. Neuroscientists call them brain insults.

After a head knock, the headaches may start along with a host of other symptoms: trouble learning, memory loss, concentration problems, behaviour problems, aggression, personality changes, etc. Some may be temporary or some may last a lifetime. Concussions do not show up on x-rays but are evident through these other signs and symptoms.

Here is one example of how brain research is changing our lives. There is a continuing debate around the world. Should headgear be compulsive for young children playing organized soccer? Neuroscience says YES. Coaches say NO. Informed parents are debating.

Brain injuries are still a mystery. But, as more is known about the brain and the general public becomes more informed, sports like boxing, football and hockey will become less popular. "Head banger sports" are _too_ dangerous! People will be less willing to put themselves, family members or their friends into positions of getting potential brain damage! The old attitude of "getting your lights knocked out" being just part of the game is total ignorance! Why take a chance. Contact sports are an endangered species.

It is obviously wise to wear a helmet to protect your head whenever necessary.

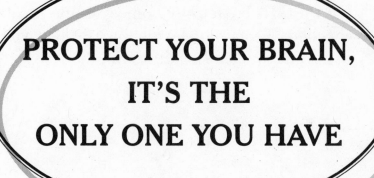

PROTECT YOUR BRAIN,
IT'S THE
ONLY ONE YOU HAVE

## 8.12  HOMOCYSTEINE TEST

Medical science has recently discovered a major factor contributing to brain breakdown, a real bad guy. Homocysteine is an amino acid produced in every cell in your body. If there is too much, it can accumulate in the blood and destroy blood vessels. Researchers say that it is a major player involved in why your intellectual abilities fail. Elevated levels increase your risk of stroke and dementia. They are also implicated as a cause of Alzheimer's disease. Excess homocysteine shrinks your brain.

The anecdote for this is inexpensive and simple. It is recommended to take B vitamins. Without B vitamins, homocysteine builds up in the blood. B's zap homocysteine.

**KEY POINT:** Get our homocysteine levels checked. Keep your levels low. Protect your self from that bad brain toxin.

# 8.13 DOWNTIME

Downtime is essential. It needs to be a top priority on everyone's "how to stay sane" list. Downtime on the job, in your daily schedule, in your overall lifestyle is an intelligent strategy you need to adopt for supporting your own wellness.

Be aware that the brain you have right now is not designed for constant input. Yet, on a daily basis, it is routinely bombarded with constant stimuli and information. Input, input, input! Snap, crackle, pop! Competing stimuli perpetually bombard your brain. We expect our brain to be 100% focused, on task all day long. We push our brain's capacity to the limits. That's not healthy.

Suppose you are trying to learn something new. It is hard to process and remember it the first time. Right? Of course, we all have experienced this many times. New meaning comes from internalizing. Therefore, other "stuff" needs to stop coming into our brain for a while! Time is required to imprint what we have just learned into our memory banks. New synapses will not form in your brain with endless competing stimuli. Learning is a complicated process. When learning new material, your brain needs breaks. It needs time to sort, file and make sense of what it is that you are trying to learn.

Purposeful downtime is crucial for a number of reasons. Your memory relies on it. If you want to keep your memory sharp then you need daily, regular downtime. Downtime gives you mental power. It allows your prefrontal cortex to filter out information, sort messages, to plan and to make decisions. It maintains a healthy brain and promotes longevity. You have less fatigue. Obviously taking an occasional break bolsters your mental performance.

"I have no time for downtime". What a cop out! Yet, that's the way we live. Here's how to put time on your side.

In the morning, most people are generally bright and sharp. But, in the afternoon, that can disappear. The genius in you has gone and you just barely think like a slug. You need to give your brain all the intelligent support it can get. The POWER SNOOZE or NAP is one of the top secrets for brain longevity and survival.

Here's how to calculate when to have a power snooze. Suppose you went to sleep at 10 pm and woke up around 6 am the next day. You would therefore be awake from 6 am to 10 pm (16 hours). The mid point of your day would be half way through (8 hours). Therefore the very best time for you to have a power snooze would be around 2 pm.

The ideal power snooze is never more than 30 minutes at the low point of the day when your brain circuits need it most. A quick snooze or rest keeps your brain from burning out. Doesn't this make sense to you? Recharge your brain batteries. I have power snoozed for most of my adult life. It's not a waste of time. No guilt for me. I need one to stay mentally sharp.

When you decide to have some have downtime, you do not need to fall asleep. The objective is to simply relax the brain and produce more alpha waves. Nothing special is needed except perhaps an alarm clock. Try darkening the room and doing some deep breathing. Some people like to listen to calming music. Your attitude should be supportive. You need to convince yourself that you are benefiting from this short downtime. If you do fall asleep, that's good. If you don't, you still benefit from lowered blood pressure, shutting down the hassles for a bit of time and rejuvenating your mental energies.

Sometimes there may not be a chance for a power snooze. You may not even like the idea of it. Your next best alternative is movement. A short walk, bending or stretching can stimulate the body out of drowsiness. Other genuine approaches include: drawing, journaling, doing a puzzle, doing a totally different mental exercise, reflecting in silence, or enjoying a cup of herbal tea. Whatever suits you is valid as long as it gives you the break you need from that constant brain input. This has to happen if you want to maintain and sustain many years of high productivity. Take some downtime everyday.

Here are three excellent brain wellness downtime activities:

1. **Palm your eyes.** This is very beneficial to relieve eyestrain and provide mental relaxation. First warm your palms by rubbing them together. Then, rest your elbows on the table. Close your eyes. Cover your eyes with your palms and practice deep breathing for a few minutes.

2. **Massage your big toes.** Reflexologists massage body points on the feet to send healing energy to the entire body. The reflex points for your brain are on the soft padded side of each big toe.

3. **Walk around barefooted.** We wear shoes most of the time all year round. Our feet don't touch the ground very often. The soles of our feet have special sensory receptors that communicate position information from our feet to the brain. These receptors are major contributors to good balance. Walk on many different surfaces to support your balance and ability to avoid falling.

# 8.14 TIME IN NATURE

People are not separate from Mother Nature. There is a great inner need to be in contact with nature. Nature renews and heals us physically, emotionally, mentally and spiritually. Nature re-energizes us and supplies our life energy. Our thoughts are raised, our health improves and our creativity flows when we visit the oceans, forests, beaches, mountains, or parks. Don't be divided from nature, stay connected.

Mother Nature is not man made. When we visit the natural world, our brain receives positive images. The pictures we view are complete. There are not fragments. Images don't flip past us at rocket speeds. Nature counter balances our chaotic, stressful and sometimes violent world. Nature supports us to be healthier and happier humans. The natural world offers unity, balance and harmony.

No time to get out into nature? Why not bring nature into your home or office? Try listening to nature music or acquire some common houseplants. They filter pollutants from our air and put some green into our living environments. NASA research scientists recommend the peace lily with its dark glossy leaves and lovely white flowers for clearing toxins. Other beneficial plants include: Chinese evergreen, English ivy, rubber plant, Boston fern, ficus and the spider plant. Grow your own fresh air. Enjoy!

## 8.15  PLAY FOR FUN

I fondly recall taking my young son to the playground to play on the slides and swings when he was about 4 years old. He was just having a great time along with five or six other kids. Me too. I was climbing and sliding right along with the whole gang. Then it happened. Right in the middle of this experience I looked up and there they were. A long somber line of parents staring at me and the kids. They resembled a row of mannequins in a store window display. What a revelation! Those parents had forgotten how to play.

Nature intended us to play so that we could develop our brains. Our experiences playing establish endless multiple pathways for learning. The more you play the more you develop your brain. Playing has other positive spinoffs by boosting your self-esteem, developing your motor skills and enhancing your problem solving skills.

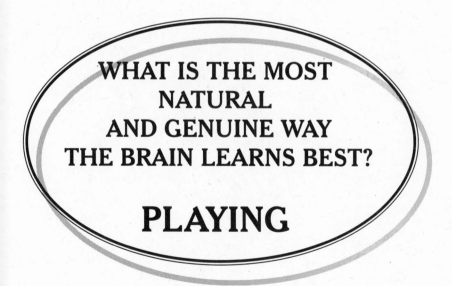

WHAT IS THE MOST
NATURAL
AND GENUINE WAY
THE BRAIN LEARNS BEST?

PLAYING

I am not referring to organized adult sports. Playing games with strict rules, competitions with winners and losers are too limiting. I am referring to just playing for the sake of playing, Play with whatever you can have fun with. There is nothing wrong with playing with toys once in a while no matter what your age is. Make time to play. Go outside and play like the kids do.

I am sure you have noticed that children have a compulsion to play. That's Nature's design. It is part of the essence of life. As adults, we have lost it. Life is mostly about work. That's the goal of society. Get a job and work. Play is not for adults because it is considered a waste of time. That's unfortunate.

Adults need to play more. Play can be the secret player in our personal success. We can all play at anything we want. There is an infinite variety of ways to play. The key points are to play with no expectations, no rewards and without any time pressures. It's not needing to be on top or being the best. Outcome should not be a factor. Playing should be the intrinsic reward itself.

Learn to play at work. Learn to work at play. Playing is a state of consciousness that sets you free. That's when your brain works best and you grow dendrites like crazy.

# 8.16 HUMOUR

A laughing brain is a healthy brain. How can humans live without laughter? Humour is a condition that helps us flourish. Laughter and good humour help bring joy into our lives.

Laughter is the perfect antidote to stress. Like exercise, laughter produces the same positive mind-body benefits. A good laugh produces the youthful hormone DHEA. DHEA comes from your adrenal glands. DHEA helps to reduce stress, give you energy and keep your brain young. Another benefit is that adrenalin production is reduced in the bloodstream. If adrenalin is produced all day long, fatigue and exhaustion are sure to follow. Adrenalin rushes are harder to handle as you age. As well, the stressful levels of cortisol are reduced with a good chuckle keeping your brain out of the fight or flight response.

When we laugh and smile we live in a more beneficial, biochemical environment. The stress chemicals are being replaced by serotonin, the mood boosting neurotransmitter. Serotonin floods your brain when you enjoy a humorous moment counter acting stress. Dopamine levels also soar.

Humour does a lot of other wonderful life supporting things for us. It protects us from the ravages of negative emotions. Laughter makes us feel good. When we feel good we are healthier, happier, work more productively and live more enjoyable lives. Laughter uplifts us from our busy life providing an escape from the rat race. Laughter is good medicine that strengthens our immune system and eases depression. Happy people are less prone to illness.

Laughter clubs are springing up around the world. Dr. Madan Kataria started the first one in India in 1995 encouraging people just to laugh for fun. His website is www.laughteryoga.com. Today there are over 5000 laughter clubs in 40 different countries.

The New Science of Happiness is a big trend in psychology today. Could laughter be one of the biggest secrets for keeping our body, mind and brain healthy? A good source of humour goes a long way in today's world.

Are you taking life too seriously? Do you sometimes have a constipated expression on your face? If so, you may need to loosen up and have a few more laughs. Invite humour into your life. Joke about yourself. After all, some of your behaviours and attitudes could be the biggest jokes of all and you wouldn't want to miss them.

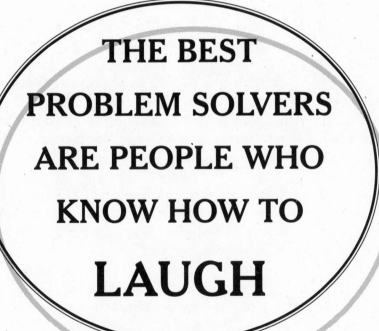

THE BEST PROBLEM SOLVERS ARE PEOPLE WHO KNOW HOW TO LAUGH

# 8.17  SLEEP SECRETS

Are you yawning throughout the day? Nodding off at the office? Low on energy? Do you get lots of sleep but still feel exhausted the next day? For me, a lack of sleep does not feel great. I can't focus and I can't think. That sucks! I know my pre-frontal cortex that I need for learning and memory is not on line. If I get enough sleep, I am efficient, productive and a happy brain owner. That's the way I want my life to be. I'm sure you do too!

Your lifestyle could be "early to bed, early to rise" or, it could be "burning the midnight oil". Regardless, imagine being wide-awake and alert all day long, every day. Knowledge is power. Here is one of the greatest brain wellness secrets revealed.

As mentioned previously, your brain works on 90-minute cycles. Your sleeping cycles are the same. Here is a very simpli-fied overview of your brain's sleep cycles.

After falling asleep, your brain would proceed to have 65 minutes of normal sleep. Then, it would have 20 minutes of REM sleep (Rapid Eye Movement or Dream State) and finish with 5 more minutes of normal sleep. This would complete one sleep cycle, 90 minutes or 1½ hours.

Uninterrupted cycles would then be:

1 sleep cycle ................ 1.5 hours
2 sleep cycles .............. 3.0 hours
3 sleep cycles .............. 4.5 hours
4 sleep cycles .............. 6.0 hours
5 sleep cycles .............. 7.5 hours
6 sleep cycles .............. 9.0 hours
7 sleep cycles .............. 10.5 hours

In the morning, you need to wake up as close as possible to the end of a sleep cycle not in the middle of one. I sleep 5 cycles. I try not to wake up after 7 hours or 8 hours because these times are not in line with the completion of 5 cycles. I have practiced this for many years with good success. I set my alarm clock for 7.5 hours and GET UP when the alarm rings. That way, I start my day the brain smart way.

When you are asleep, the motor cortex system of your brain is shut down. If you wake up in REM sleep before the end of a cycle, you are often lifeless, drowsy and lack get up and go. The reason is because your motor cortex hasn't started up yet. Train yourself to wake up at 6 hours or 7 ½ or 9 hours when the sleep cycle has ended. You can't get exactly to the minute but as close as you can to those times is the secret.

I'm sure you have seen an endless number of tired looking people in the morning. If you can get your sleep patterns in line with the brain's natural rhythms, you will reap the benefits. It's better than caffeine. Of course there are lots of exceptions. Nursing mothers can't follow these patterns. Extremely stressed individuals can't either. Shift work makes it very difficult to follow. However, understanding how the brain normally sleeps is simple and easy. Applying it can be the challenge.

Here are some additional helpful tips for sleeping well and recharging your brain as suggested by sleep experts. Your best sleeping hours are 2 hours before midnight. Go to sleep and wake up at the same time every day. That will put you into a healthy sleep pattern – the body likes sleep regularity. Don't do strenuous exercise just before going to sleep. If you are not sleepy, worries are haunting you or your thoughts are too active, you need to slow down the brain stimulation. Neuroscientists say we need to BORE the brain down. So if you read a suspense novel, horror story or watch the news just before going to bed, your brain will be stimulated. It's better to browse a textbook or something that is not very interesting. So reading, listening to relaxing music, going for a leisurely walk, stretching, having a hot bath, or drinking a cup of herbal tea will set the stage for sleeping.

Alcohol is not recommended as a sleep aid. Coffee has benefits during the day but not for supporting good sleep. Coffee reduces the quality and quantity of sleep. Thousands upon thousands of people take sleeping pills. Avoid the insomnia epidemic. I suggest that you get very well educated on the pros and cons of using medications. Seek other alternatives.

Finally, it is highly recommended to sleep in a room that is as dark as possible. Turn off the lights. When you are lying in bed in darkness, the brain tells the body to shut down and go to sleep. Also, sleeping in a cool room is better than a warm room, if possible. Around 16-18 degrees Celsius seems to be the best temperature as the body is not adjusting to being too hot or too cold. Finally, sleep with an open window if you can. If your bedroom is like a cool, quiet, dark cave, the stage is set for a positive sleep.

**WARNING: YOUR BRAIN IS NOT WIRED FOR GETTING ONLY 6 HOURS OF SLEEP EVERY NIGHT.**
**IN THE LONG RUN, THIS WILL EVENTUALLY IMPAIR YOUR BRAIN FUNCTION.**

# 8.18 CREATIVE VISUALIZATION

Visualization is an awesome, personal tool. It's easy. It takes only a few minutes to do. Athletes, musicians, actors, public speakers and countless others have practiced visualization techniques for years to improve their performance. You could too. It works. Brain imaging machines provide scans that prove it.

Your brain is a powerful organ. If you imagined yourself doing a task, the neurons in your brain would light up the same as if you were really doing it. By engaging in mental rehearsal, your brain establishes a new pattern before it actually happens. You can therefore influence your performance on any task, skill or activity by creating it in your mind ahead of time. Every time you visualize it, you get better and better.

Here is an example. You want a challenge in your life so you decide to hike up a local mountain. You have never done this before and you are concerned it may be beyond your limits but you are determined to succeed. Here's how to use your personal inbuilt success device. It's best done in a quiet place with closed eyes.

First, think about hiking up the mountain. Create mental images about it. Your brain has millions of stored pictures already. Hook into this gigantic blueprint that will display every thing you know about hiking (maps, trails, boots, equipment, rain gear, food etc...). Secondly, visualize yourself with no problems reaching the summit. See yourself climbing up higher and higher. Create images of all the sights, sounds, and feelings that you would experience on the way up. Finally, visualize yourself standing on the top of the mountain. You made it. Make your visualization pictures colourful, intense, exciting and full of details. You have mentally rehearsed your climb before you actually did it. You set up the correct program and your brain did the rest. Creative visualization is a mental warm-up supporting your success. It is a super compliment for any activity you can think of.

# 8.19 STRESS BREAKERS

Are you planning for an early brain burnout? Is stress destroying your brain? People vary tremendously in many ways including how they respond to stress. Our brains face daily challenges it's not designed to deal with. Rush hour line-ups, deadlines, on going multitasking mean you need to be prepared for how to deal with them because your brain isn't. Stress takes your 'Captain' off line. We can deal with a wild animal trying to eat us but not with the mountains of paperwork on the desk. Modern day stress is bad for your brain. Chronic stress means premature aging of your brain. It's called **neuroerosion** or slow brain death. No one wants day in day out stress to eat away at his/her brainpower. But, it does!

Stress management is critical if you want to be well. You have to be very smart indeed, to deal with stress wisely. Whether you experience chronic, unrelenting stress or occasional stress, you need to be aware of how it affects you. Otherwise, you may fall victim to the many chronic lifestyle diseases that our hunter-gatherer ancestors never had.

Here are some basic approaches:

**1. Don't be in denial.** If you are always low on energy, can't find enthusiasm in anything or have no more confidence, these may be burn out signs. Do not ignore the signs.

**2. You must have a relaxation technique.** Again, this is not an option. It is critical for your survival to have personal control measures. You may not be able to manipulate outside stressors but you can regulate what goes on inside of you.

**3. Deep breathe your stress away.** Breathing is a good thing to do. Get lots of oxygen into your brain.

**4. You don't have to do every thing.** Cut back; learn to say

"No". Have you noticed that busy people are always given more to do because they seem to get things done? Don't commit to doing something right away. Take some time to think about it first. Be wise about your commitments.

**5. Get lots of sleep.** It's hard to cope with stress if you are always tired. Why live with decreased brain function? If you are challenged with insomnia, seek professional help.

**6. Aerobic exercise has been repeatedly proven to reduce stress.** It remains one of the best possible ways to get stress relief. Walking is the simplest brain smart activity.

**7. Yawning is the brain's signal for more oxygen.** (See 4.5 Brain Gym)

**8. Meditation has a long list of positive benefits.** Researchers are showing how meditation directly affects the brain in positive ways. Meditation has been practiced for thousands of years all over the world by countless millions of people.

**9. Avoid excess that destroys your brain.** Overwork, no vacation time, too much coffee, too many alcoholic drinks, smoking, drug use are all undesirable habits for coping with stress and life's challenges.

**10. Eat well.** Enjoy nutritious foods whenever you can. Eat lots of fiber, reduce your fat, eat less salt and munch down those antioxidant foods. Supplements like B vitamins can be effective support during stressful times.

**11. Worrying threatens your brain.** Even an imaginary threat is perceived by your brain as if the threat were actually happening. Your brain is powerful. Freaking out ahead of time can trigger your brain into stress response. Why worry so much?

**12. Try not to get too emotional.** Take control of your

emotions to help you stay mentally sharp.

**13. If depression is an issue, get help!** Support from a trained professional can boost your self-esteem and help you get back on track.

**14. If you are always racing the clock, try these on your 25th hour:** bubble bath, sauna, massage, aromatherapy, good music, relaxation tapes, nature sounds, walk in the park, watch a funny movie, or just invest some quality time on yourself.

**15. Be happy! Feel good!** Do what you want to do in life. Your life can be heaven or hell on earth. Make sure your brain is full of serotonin and dopamine instead of cortisol. You are the conductor of your own life's symphony. Play a great tune.

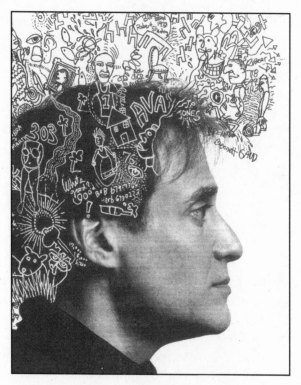

How to Improve Memory, Time, June 12, 2000.

# 8.20  THE MEMORY SOLUTION

Your memory is not a thing. It is a living process. Your memory is dynamic by nature. It changes and evolves constantly as new experiences and information are added to it. Your memory is an extraordinarily complex process depending upon one single, critical skill.

There are many, many books and improvement guides to help you with your memory. There are hundreds of sites on the Web. Videos, games and expert opinions are springing up everywhere. Memory is a hot topic so products are really starting to flood the market. It is my experience that buying technical memory books or surfing the net may not do you much good. I have taught memory skills to teachers, students and the general public for over 20 years. I teach people one fundamental skill and once you are aware of it, you will not need to spend a single penny on improving your memory. You have everything you need already.

As time passes, memory is the first faculty to go. I hope you will see fit to try this memory solution before that happens. I wish to offer you some practical hands on advice. There are no quick fixes. Miracles are unlikely. Please realize that your memory is not perfect. It can fade over time. That's a fact for all of us. Don't worry about doing championship memory training techniques to get a reliable memory. You simply have to learn how to **pay attention**.

For some people, this may sound very boring or dry. If you would rather have a quick fix, a one-a-day pill, or a complex scientific analysis, forget it! The answer is before you. **Paying attention is the creative player for owning a workable memory**. It's a fact that there cannot be any memory at all without some degree of attention. The accuracy of your memory and the strength of your recall depend upon how well you can **concentrate**. If you are paying attention, you are concentrating. If you are not paying attention, you are not concentrating and there goes your memory. The bottom line is this. If you start to cultivate your powers of attention, your memory will improve and strengthen. Exercise it, little by little, day by day and you will be able to remember more and accomplish more. Train your mind to be attentive.

**The first tip is to learn to do one thing at a time without thinking about anything else.** Do what is before you and then move onto the next thing. Since the brain can only do one thing at a time, it is very difficult to be doing one thing while thinking of something completely different. Get into this most critical habit. Your brain performance and output will greatly improve. Do one thing at a time. Your aging memory depends on it.

How do you practice keeping your concentration? You know as well as everyone else, that if you are interested in an object, it will hold your attention. Therefore, begin by practicing with an ordinary, uninteresting object. This requires a much greater effort. **Willpower** is called for. It is willpower that is behind the ability to pay attention and hence remember.

First Round of Practice. Tell your memory that you are going to play a game. Pick up any household object and place it before you, a pencil for example. You want to study this object. What is its shape, size, weight, colour, model name, use, purpose, smell, value, etc. and dozens of other characteristics? Analyze it, take it apart and reduce it to its simplest parts. The more your attention is fixed, the deeper the memory imprint. Then write all your observations down. Spend at least 25-30 minutes doing your observation. That long? Yes, stick with it.

Next day, check out the same pencil again writing down any additional impressions that you have found. This will strengthen your attention because you have to will yourself to focus on it and this will deepen your memory of it. You will get better and better at doing this. Do it with a friend to add interest. Sounds very simple and unexciting but it works.

Second Round of Practice. The next level of attention building escalates from the first. Pick a display window in a store. Walk past just glancing at the contents. Note what you saw and write the details down. You will miss many things on the first attempt. But, next time you will improve. Have someone do this with you. You can play at this anywhere at any time. Use rooms, photographs, people, magazines or any scene that is available. With these simple games, you are undoing bad memory habits based on a failure to focus and concentrate. You need to use your natural willpower to cultivate your powers of attention. This takes practice, practice, and more practice.

Finally, by putting new interest into improving your attention, your memory will improve. Your memory problems and concerns will gradually diminish. Invest in your own survival. Help yourself. There is no real cost other than time well spent and a whole lot of effort. It's not such a mystery after all.

# CHAPTER 9

# The Critical Requirements

I hope this never happens to you. It may happen at any time or at any age to any one of us. One day in the future, a thought explodes in your head like a thunderbolt. This flash of light will shock you to pieces. You are losing it! Yes, you were an intelligent, capable and self-sustaining individual. Not any more. Your brain is decaying and you haven't even been aware of it. You have been living unconsciously for years totally oblivious about your brainpower slipping away on you. Could the game be up?

# 9.1  RETIRE WISELY

Some people are so busy with their work these days, they can hardly imagine a time when they will have to quit. Others, packing 40 extra pounds in a widening paunch, view their fast approaching retirement date with helpless panic. The mandatory retirement age has just been cancelled in Canada. So, you don't have to quit at age 65 if you don't want to. This has a lot of benefits for the country as a whole. But, most Canadians will eventually have to leave their full time employment. **Warning, be very careful of the following:**

**Retirement:** withdrawal from one's position or occupation, or from active working life.

NEVER RETIRE! Never, ever dream of a life of total leisure and pleasure. That is a big mistake. If you are going to end your working career, always have something else ready to replace it with. Reappraise your future carefully. Don't fall for the trap "I'll deal with it when the time comes." This huge shift in energy and change in life can be a bombshell if you are not ready. Depression can result. The brain can shut down. Too much idle time puts you in front of the TV. Instead, keep active with whatever interests you. Endless new options are open to you: new careers, new directions, part-time job, job sharing, volunteering, retraining, collecting, hobbies, etc. To age successfully, you need to be productive. Keep occupied and active until your very last days. This will help your brain stay vital and alive. Engage your intellect and support your brain health as well as your mental well being. Plan to keep on being productive.

**Remaining independent** is on the top of the list for the brain's wellness success strategies. Working well into old age will support this great dream we should all strive for. This, in my opinion, is the most significant issue to consider in your brain wellness program. Escape from **dependency** for as long as you can.

## 9.2  ATTITUDE IS EVERYTHING

Your own attitude can be a poison or an elixir. What we think is what we get. Negative thoughts and negative feelings promote disharmony and disease. Dark thoughts, negative labels, blaming, criticism, predicting the worst are your enemies. "I've got a bad memory." "I'll never remember that." "I must be getting old, my memory is going." Exorcise your own demons.

Focus on the positive. Focus on beneficial, uplifting supportive thoughts. Count your blessings. Be grateful. An attitude of gratitude floods you with feel good endorphins. Everything you do in life has a thought that precedes it. Keep those thoughts positive. Self-discipline and self-control are essential qualities rallying around your ability to think. Your future depends upon your thoughts. Old attitudes need to be renovated, thrown out, renewed. Create a new reality for yourself. Affirm: "Everyday in every way, my brain is getting better and better". As you think, so you are!

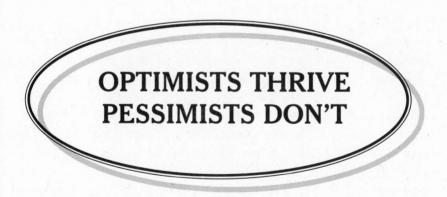

OPTIMISTS THRIVE
PESSIMISTS DON'T

# 9.3 YOUR PERSONAL VIRTUES

The most prodigious effort of your life is to learn how to play the game of brain wellness. At our current stage of evolution, humans are endlessly striving for possessions. Possessions and money are valued above all else. Unfortunately, spiritual values have been pushed into the background. Help is needed on the brain wellness path.

Keeping in the right direction may be challenging. Keeping a clear mind may also be difficult. Perseverance and a sustained effort are the secrets. Systematically plodding away with your brain wellness plan will bring you success. Keep on keeping on. Existing within each one of us are many inherent qualities. Call forth these potentials if you need them.

**Acceptance.** What is, is! You are who you are at this moment. Accept yourself and your life without judgment. You have strengths and weaknesses. Good decisions have been made as well as bad ones over your lifetime. No one is perfect. Gratefully accept yourself and your present situation regardless of your age.

Acceptance is not an easy virtue to acquire. You may need to push your pride out of the way to overcome denial. For example, if you claim that you don't have a problem paying attention, honestly ask someone you live with. You may get a very different answer. Focus on what you need to do. You now know that smoking cigarettes is a proven brain killer. Make an effort for your own health to cut back and hopefully you may be able to quit. If you are overweight, exercise. If you are a violent video game addict, get a new hobby. If you can't get going in the morning without jump-starting your brain with coffee, try something else. The solution is this. If you know that certain activities that you do are harmful to your brain, accept that fact and change your habits. Acceptance doesn't mean giving up. It means to pay attention and take appropriate action.

**Courage**. Courage is needed to transform undesirable habits in your personality. Always working too much, cut back your hours. No time for your kids, find time. Too many things on the go, set new priorities or let something go.

Courage overcomes fear. Fear holds us all back. If you decide that you are no longer going to do something, go for it. Instead of watching three hours of television every night, exercise or get an interesting hobby. If you decide junk food is no longer for you, don't eat it. If you are sick of being tired, get more sleep even though your friends want to keep on partying. It takes courage to run counter to the opinions and wishes of others. Courage will keep you from getting sidetracked from the path of wellness. If you vow to overcome destructive habits, terrific. Take heart. The courage you need lies within.

**THE SERENITY PRAYER**
**God grant me the serenity to accept**
**the things I cannot change;**
**courage to change the things I can;**
**and the wisdom to know the difference.**

**Forgiveness**. Forgiveness is certainly one of mankind's winning attributes. We have the ability to forget the past and to move forward. If we desire to, we can let go of old mistakes, policies, judgments, choices, etc. Recognize we all make mistakes. Don't get caught living for years with old hatreds. It's exhausting. What huge benefits can occur if you approach life with more love and forgiveness! Forgive yourself for being a brain abuser. Forgive yourself for years of brain neglect. Let go of the unpleasant past and move into a brighter future.

**Patience**. Patience is perhaps the greatest virtue of them all. It provides great personal power. Years of bad habits have consequences. Reversing brain damage from drug and alcohol abuse will not occur overnight. Burn out can take years to recover from. Hypertension and stress eat away at brain cells placing people permanently in survival mode. Also, time is needed for the brain to grow new circuits after a brain injury or a stroke. If you are patient, anxiety and fear are easier to cope with.

If you are always in a hurry, you probably won't have much patience. Your viewpoint will probably remain the same. It will be difficult to find your vision. Patience is not passive. Patience helps you fight your battles. In spite of all your adversaries, patience gives you the strength to try, to strive, to dare. True patience is the joy of watching your memory slowly improve. True patience is experiencing the brain fog lifting. Patience will give you your victories. It's reclaiming your ability to focus again. It's about knowing where your keys are all the time and knowing what each key does. Patience will brace you up to detach from your loss of brainpower and stay tuned to your wellness goals. Patience, and brain smarts go together.

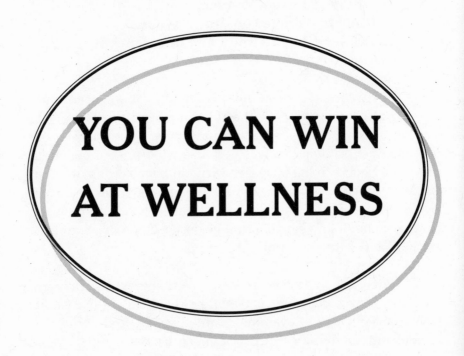

# YOU CAN WIN AT WELLNESS

# 9.4 EMBRACE CHANGE

The secrets for brain wellness have been revealed to you. One of the basic facts of life is this. Your brain will age, that is a 100% guarantee, but be grateful because practical, helpful solutions are readily available.

There is one missing piece to the whole puzzle of brain wellness that completes the picture. **Change!**

Change is the only constant in your life. Life is characterized by impermanence. We must change! You will change whether you want to or not. Your power lies in your gift of choice. If you choose to resist change, stress, pain or suffering will likely manifest. If you choose to embrace change, you can transform yourself more easily and peacefully.

Here are some signposts indicating that you may be resisting change in your life. Physically you may get sick or manifest a disease. Emotionally you could have trouble with bitterness, hatred or intolerance. Mentally, you could have problems with rigidity, narrow mindedness or stubbornness. Here's the smart solution. You need to alter yourself because maybe what you are thinking or how you are behaving is causing the problem. So, if you can change, you can help solve the problem.

There is no use worrying all the time about getting Alzheimer's disease. Your fears could be getting the best of you. You are possibly afraid because you just don't know. You hear and imagine all kinds of dreadful stuff. The general public is fearful. The general public is ignorant about brain health as well! Break away from that mind set. Don't believe the old myths. If you focus on decline, expect decline, you'll get it!

Lose your fears. Trust the universe. You can overcome fear of the unknown by **focusing on a higher purpose**. That is the antidote. What are you really good at? What is your passion? What is your gift to the world? Without a sense of purpose your contribution is hampered. Focus on your purpose as a human being and your resistance to change will evaporate.

As well, being attached to the past triggers fear of change. I find it very sad to be around people who are always talking about the past. They are frozen in time. It is far healthier to be focused in the present moment. Do not allow yourself to be attached to the past. It is more intelligent and productive to be fixed on the present! Leave the past and move ahead because that is where excitement and new visions exist. Let go. Welcome change. Create change. Embrace change! Escape from your old habits because they just might be killing you. Invite the unexpected. Make your life more interesting. Your brain will love it!

Tragedies and losses need to be overcome along the way. People you know are going to die and grief can materialize. Extended grief kills neurons. Mourning is a very draining emotion and can rob you of your energy. Attention is focused on what is lost. Overcoming it is a great challenge and can take time but it must be accomplished. Healing has to occur.

Consider this advice seriously. If you lose a friend, make a new one. As well, have friends and acquaintances besides your partner or significant other.

If your perception of reality is poor, fix it. Perhaps you are getting sick of being lethargic. Brain fatigue has become a way of life. Your brain screams for oxygen but your mind says, "forget it". You are always losing stuff and spend time looking for things. "Oh, well." A malnourished brain resides in your skull but a can of pop and a bag of chips will do. Life just seems to drain your brain. Your life style sucks! Time to change. You owe it to yourself.

But, what are people like? Faced with knowing that they have to change something, they so often get busy proving that there is no need to. Overcome this resistance. One of the very best things that the brain does constantly is **adapt**. It possesses a phenomenal ability to change. You do too. Your own innate knowledge and wisdom are freely capable of supporting you to change. You have the power to alter your own reality and control your own destiny.

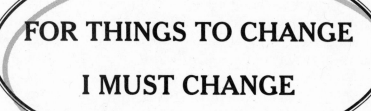 **KEY POINT:** Your greatest personal power lies in the ability to make small changes on a daily basis because the brain does not like giant paradigm shifts. Those small changes are what will make the biggest difference to your brain wellness in the long run.

## FOR THINGS TO CHANGE

## I MUST CHANGE

# 9.5  YES, YOU CAN!

As a brain coach, I am personally not the least interested in getting swept up by the fast approaching tidal wave of brain deterioration and mental dysfunction. I want to stay mentally sharp until my life is over. I know that a healthy brain means a better life. I would rather live in peace than in a constant state of fear, anxiety and stress. Can I do this? Yes, I can. So can you!

Look forward to continuously enhancing your brainpower. Avoid the battered, beleaguered brain syndrome. Escape from an unclear brain and recover to a world of clarity. Maintain a valuable, serviceable brain by staying productive and remaining healthy. Make it happen. Pursue a life of excellence and follow your dreams. Dreams are real. The knowledge, direction and the tools are yours to use. The time is now. You're the 'Captain' and the Coach so write your own script. You can do it. <u>Yes</u>, **you can!**

It's easy to recommend changing things but as you well know, it's more difficult to enact them. New ideas take time. Whether you are a young brain, baby boomer brain or senior brain, it's very easy to get overwhelmed in today's complex world! Make time! Brain wellness requires you to put your best foot forward. Brain training takes effort!

My best advice would be to start with a few of the sure bets. Start with meeting the basic biological requirements of the brain: regular exercise, proper sleep and good nutrition. Pick a few brain boosters and start to practise. Remember, that maintaining brain fitness means you have to <u>work</u> at it. Persistence is needed.

As a general rule, people are lazy. Bad habits are easy to learn and take less energy and effort than good habits. If people dealt with their emotions or challenges in life, perhaps they wouldn't need to overeat, smoke, drink alcohol or escape in a host of other ways.

Your thoughts are your habits and yet, your thoughts can be used as tools to make any changes you wish. Knowing and applying this knowledge can give you genuine personal power. Your thoughts can create good habits and can change bad habits. Our characters are really a collection of repeated habits and it's by repeating positive habits that we can reform our character. Choose to think like this. "My memory is getting better and better." "I am growing my brain all the time." "I am creating more brain power, every day in every way." Positive affirmations like these become new beneficial habits. Your choice of positive thoughts can become the foundation of your brain wellness program. As well, affirmations strengthen the good habits you already have.

Commit to a few new brain boosting habits and stick with them. Believe in your brain. Believe that it is strong and reliable. Use your imagination. Visualize blood flowing to your brain. Create ways to help yourself maintain a youthful and dynamic brain for the rest of your life. You cannot afford to lose the brain wellness game. Brain problems happen gradually over time so be proactive today or face your fate tomorrow. As a brain coach, don't forget to go out the door every day for the rest of your life with your....

# COMMON SENSE

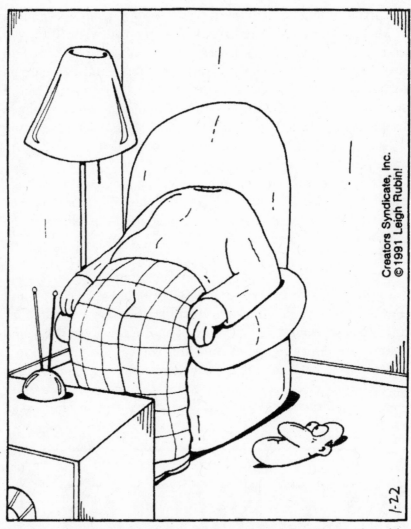

Quite suddenly and without warning, Herb fell victim to the old
adage, "If you don't use it, you lose it."

Rubes by Leigh Rubin

# 10

# Ten Top Brain Wellness Secrets

As a brain coach, here are your first-rate practical strategies for enhancing your brain and avoiding deterioration. They all work together as a wellness team providing you with the benefits you need. Cross train your brain just like you would cross train your body.

**1. Prevention.** You are personally responsible for maintaining your own brain wellness. You now have the knowledge to enhance, protect and maintain optimum brain functioning for your entire lifetime. Brain decline does not have to be inevitable. Keep your master organ healthy.

**2. Exercise supports neurogenesis.** A sedentary lifestyle is irrational. Avoid being paralyzed by today's sluggish modern life. Regular activity gets lots of fresh blood and oxygen to every neuron in your brain as well as creating new neurons. Stay active everyday. Exercise keeps dementia away.

**3. A brain sustaining diet is critical for brain wellness.** Make healthy food choices. Eat only cell friendly foods. Support yourself with supplements and herbs. Omega 3 oil is indispensable. Water is essential for concentration and mental alertness.

**4. Get enough sleep so that you are alert and energetic everyday.** Daily brainpower needs a good sleep every night. Your overall brainpower and memory rely on it.

**5. Practice some form of de-stress activity.** Stress kills brain cells. Chronic stress alters the chemistry of your brain promoting free radical production and accelerating aging.

**6. Grow dendrites.** Keep on learning. Education is a lifelong occupation. The brain loves novelty and challenge not endless predictable routines. Brain fitness requires learning something new all the time to support plasticity.

**7. Protect your fragile brain.** Wear a helmet if needed. Avoid substances that poison or destroy your neurons.

**8. Remain socially active.** Stimulating relationships, friendships and partnerships are really important. We have a natural desire for these interactions. Keep your social brain healthy.

**9. Pay attention**. Maintain what you already have. If you are losing brainpower, do something about it before things get progressively worse. There are many simple and inexpensive things you can do. Ask yourself, "Am I living and working in a brain compatible environment?"

**10. Experience life.** Live all you can and avoid doing nothing. Brain wellness and longevity require embracing change, striving to maintain your independence and living your life to its fullest.

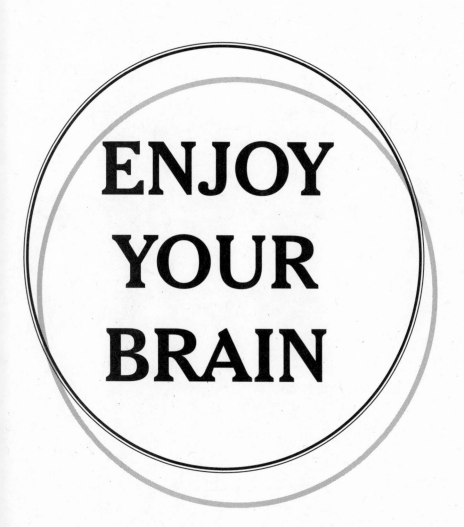

ENJOY YOUR BRAIN

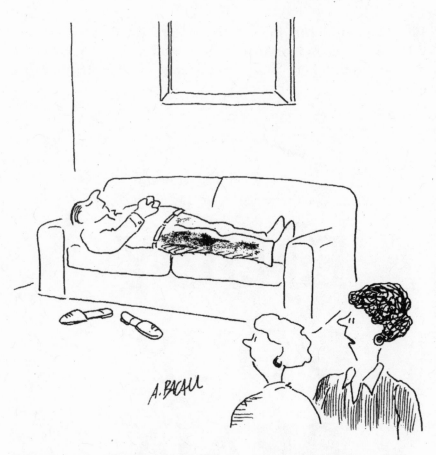

"He spent two thousand dollars on gym equipment and all he ever exercises is caution."

Cartoonist: Aaron Bacall

# RESOURCES

## Books

Amen, Daniel G., M.D. *Making A Good Brain Great*. Harmony Books, New York, NY, 2005.

Amen, Daniel G., M.D. *Change Your Brain Change Your Life*. Three Rivers Press, New York, NY, 1998.

Benton, David. *Food For Thought*. Penguin Books, London, 1996.

Blaylock, Russell L., M.D. *Excitotoxins The Taste that Kills*. Health Press, Santa Fe, New Mexico, 1997.

Buzan, Tony. *Make the Most of Your Mind*. Fireside/Simon & Schuster, New York, NY, 1988.

Buzan, Tony with Buzan, Barry *The Mindmap Book Radiant Thinking*. BBC Books, London, 1995.

Buzan, Tony. *Use Both Sides Of Your Brain*. Plume/Penguin Group, New York, NY, 1989.

Campbell, Don. *The Mozart Effect*. Avon Books, Inc./HarperCollins Publishers, Inc., New York, NY, 1997.

Carper, Jean. *Stop Aging Now! The Ultimate Plan For Staying Young & Reversing The Aging Process*. HarperCollins Publishers, Inc., New York, NY, 1995.

Carper, Jean. *Your Miracle Brain*. HarperCollins Publishers, Inc., New York, NY, 2000.

Crook III, Thomas H., Ph.D. and Adderly, Brenda, M.H.A. *The Memory Cure*. Pocket Books, New York, NY, 1998.

Dennison, Paul E., Ph.D. and Dennison, Gail E. *Brain Gym*

*Teacher's Edition Revised.* Educational Kinesiology Foundation, Ventura, CA, 1994.

Dennison, Gail E., Dennison, Paul E., Ph.D. and Teplitz, Jerry V., J.D., Ph.D. *Brain Gym for Business Instant Brain Boosters for On-the-Job Success.* Edu-Kinestetics, Inc., Ventura, CA, 1994

Dryden, Gordon and Vos, Jeannette, Ed.D. *The Learning Revolution.* Jalmar Press, Rolling Hills Estates, California, 1994.

Goleman, Daniel. *Emotional Intelligence.* Bantam Books/Division of Bantam Doubleday Dell Publishing Group, Inc., New York, NY, 1995.

Graci, Sam. *The Path To Phenomenal Health.* John Wiley & Sons Canada, Ltd., Mississauga, ON, 2005.

Hannaford, Carla, Ph.D. *Smart Moves Why Learning Is Not All In Your Head.* Great Ocean Publishers, Atlanta, Georgia, 1995.

Katz, Lawrence C., Ph.D. & Rubin, Manning. *Keep Your Brain Alive 83 Neurobic Exercises.* Workman Publishing Company, Inc., New York, NY, 1999.

Kawashima, Ryuta. *Train Your Brain.* Kumon Publishing Co., Ltd., Tokyo, Japan, 2001.

Kenyon, Tom, M.A. *Brain States.* United States Publishing, Naples, FL, 1994.

Khalsa, Dharma Singh, M.D. with Stauth, Cameron. *Brain Longevity The Breakthrough Medical Program that Improves Your Mind and Memory.* Warner Books, Inc., New York, NY, 1997.

Kotulak, Ronald. *Inside The Brain Revolutionary Discoveries*

*Of How The Mind Works.* Andrews McMeel Publishing, Kansas City, Missouri, 1996.

Leviton, Richard. *Brain Builders! A Lifelong Guide To Sharper Thinking, Better Memory, And An Age-Proof Mind.* Reward Books/Penguin Group(USA), Inc., New York, NY, 1995.

Lorrayne, Harry & Lucas, Jerry. *The Memory Book.* Ballantine Books/A Division of Random House, Inc., New York, NY, 1974.

McKhann, Guy, M.D. and Albert, Marilyn, Ph.D. *Keep Your Brain Young The Complete Guide to Physical and Emotional Health and Longevity.* John Wiley & Sons, Inc., Hoboken, New Jersey, 2002.

Markowitz, Karen, M.A. and Jensen, Eric, M.A. *The Great Memory Book.* The Brain Store Inc., San Diego, CA, 1999.

Michaud, Ellen, Wild, Russell. and the editors of Prevention Magazine. *Boost Your Brain Power A Total Program To Sharpen Your Thinking and Age-Proof Your Mind.* Rodale Press, Inc., Emmaus, PA, 1991.

Nelson, Aaron P., Ph.D. with Gilbert, Susan. *The Harvard Medical School Guide To Achieving Optimal Memory.* McGraw-Hill, New York, NY, 2005.

Ostrander, Sheila and Schroeder, Lynn. *Superlearning.* Delta/The Confucian Press, Dell, New York, NY, 1979.

Pelton, Ross, R.Ph., Ph.D. with Clarke Pelton, Taffy. *Mind Food & Smart Pills A Sourcebook For The Vitamins, Herbs & Drugs That Can Increase Intelligence, Improve Memory, & Prevent Brain Aging.* Doubleday/Division of Bantam Doubleday Dell Publishing Group, Inc., New York, NY, 1989.

Perlmutter, David, M.D. and Colman, Carol. *The Better Brain*

*Book.* Riverhead Books/Penguin Group (USA) Inc., New York, NY, 2004.

Restak, Richard, M.D. *Mozart's Brain and the Fighter Pilot Unleashing Your Brain's Potential.* Harmony Books/Crown Publishing Group, New York, NY, 2001.

Restak, Richard, M.D. *Older & Wiser How To Maintain Peak Mental Ability for As Long As You Live.* Simon & Schuster, New York, NY, 1997.

Restak, Richard, M.D. *The Secret Life Of The Brain.* Dana Press and Joseph Henry Press, Washington, D.C., 2001.

Schwartz, George R., M.D. *In Bad Taste  The MSG Syndrome.* Health Press/Division of Healing Research, Inc., Santa Fe, New Mexico, 1988.

Victoroff, Jeff, M.D. *Saving Your Brain  The Revolutionary Plan To Boost Brain Power, Improve Memory, and Protect Yourself Against Aging and Alzheimer's.* Bantam Dell/Division of Random House, Inc., New York, NY, 2002.

Warren, Tom. *Beating Alzheimer's  A Step Towards Unlocking The Mysteries Of Brain Diseases.* Avery Publishing Group, Inc., Garden City Park, New York, NY, 1991.

**General Reference Books**

Bloom, Floyd E., M.D., Beal, M. Flint, M.D. and Kupfer, David K., M.D. *The Dana Guide To Brain Health  A Practical Family Reference From Medical Experts.* The Dana Foundation, New York, NY, 2006.

Howard, Pierce J., Ph.D. *The Owners Manual For The Brain Third Edition  Everyday Applications from Mind-Brain Research.* Bard Press, Austin, Texas, March 2006.

## Magazines/Newsletters

Life Extension Magazine, www.lef.org

Nutrition Action Health Letter, circa@cspinet.org

Brain Work, The Neuroscience Newsletter, rtalley@dana.org (free)

Neuroscience For Kids, chudler@u.washington.eda (free)

Alive Magazine, www.alive.com (free at Health Food Stores)

Brain Fitness News, www.positscience.com (free)

## Brain Building Programs

Brain Fitness Program 2.0, Posit Science Corp., (www.positscience.com)

Brain Age, Nintendo Co., (www.brainage.com)

Happy Neuron, QUIXIT Inc., (www.happyneuron.com)

MyBrainTrainer.com, MyBrainTrainer LLC. (www.mybraintrainer.com)

MindFit, CogniFit Ltd., (www.cognifit.com)

## Website Suggestions

**Research**
www.dana.org  (Excellent technical site)
www.brainresearch.com
www.sciam.com
www.neurosci.nature.com  (Technical articles)
www.sfn.org  (Society for Neuroscience)

## General/Educational
www.learningconnection.ca
www.brain.com
www.mypyramid.gov (Nutrition)
www.sharpbrains.com (Brain Fitness)
www.youramazingbrain.org (General)
www.thebrainmatters.org (Health)
www.brainwaveprograms.com (Health, fun)

## Brain Images/Brain Atlas
www.midworkspress.com
www.brainplace.com
www.brainmaps.org

## Puzzles/Games
www.thinks.com
www.puzzles.com

## Video Series
The Secret Life Of The Brain (Baby's Brain, Child's Brain, Teenage Brain, Adult Brain and Aging Brain),
www.pbs.org/brain
The Brain Our Universe Within, Discovery Channel

## Wellness
National Sleep Foundation, www.sleepfoundation.org
Alzheimer Society Of Canada, www.alzheimer.ca
1-800-616-8816
National Institute Of Health, www.nih.gov

# Note Page

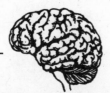

# Note Page

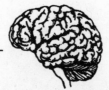

# Note Page

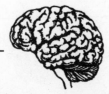

# Note Page

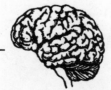

# About the Author

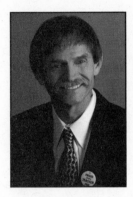

Gary Anaka is a Learning Assistance Specialist with over 30 quality years of teaching experience in regular classroom instruction, ESL and gifted enrichment. He is a Study Skills expert and a Brain Gymnastics Coach. Since 1997, he has worked as a Brain-Based Learning facilitator offering Professional Development to new and veteran teachers. He specializes in family workshops – mom, dad and their children learning together as a family. Gary is the author of Your Magical Brain: How It Learns Best – a resource book for teachers and parents. Copies can be obtained from laorder@bctf.ca.

Currently, Gary also presents seminars, workshops and keynotes supporting Brain Wellness for workplaces, special interest groups, corporations, seniors and the general public. His energetic and lively sessions offer genuine and meaningful help to support people of all ages to learn about the brain and how to maintain Brain Wellness. He is a motivational teacher whose engaging sessions have been called, both professionally and personally, life changing.

## Trainings facilitated by Gary Anaka

**Brain Wellness: The Secrets For Longevity** – All audiences interested in Brain Wellness. Genuine practical help is offered providing hope and optimism for the future of everyone's brain.

**Brain-Based Learning** – Pro-D for veteran and new teachers at the school and district level with a focus on how the brain learns best by modeling it.

**How The Brain Learns Best** – Family workshops for elementary, middle and secondary schools.

**How To Grow The Child's Brain** – Professional development for early childhood educators and parents.

**Help For An Aging Memory** – Practical support for maintaining memory as you age using a fun, interactive games approach.

Gary can be contacted at ganaka@telus.net. A full scope of his work can be viewed at www.braincoach.ca.